THE WAYSIDERS

The WAYSIDERS

READING AND THE DYSLEXIC CHILD

BY

R. M. N. Crosby, M.D.

WITH ROBERT A. LISTON

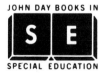

JOHN DAY BOOKS IN

S E

SPECIAL EDUCATION

THE JOHN DAY COMPANY / NEW YORK

1 2 3 4 5 6 7 8 9 10

Library of Congress Cataloging in Publication Data

Crosby, Robert M   N   1920–
   The waysiders.

   Bibliography: p.
   Includes index.
   1. Dyslexia.   I. Liston, Robert A., joint author.
II. Title.   [DNLM: 1. Dyslexia.   2. Reading.
WL340 C949w]
LB1050.5.C74   1976   371.9′14   76-12222
ISBN 0-381-98290-4

The authors gratefully acknowledge that permission to
use material was given by the following:

DAVID P. AUSUBEL: *The Psychology of Meaningful
   Verbal Learning;* Grune & Stratton, Inc., New York,
   1963.

ROGER BROWN: *Words and Things;* Free Press, Glencoe, Illinois, 1958.

D. O. HEBB: *The Organization of Behavior;* John
   Wiley & Sons, New York, 1949.

DONALD D. DURRELL: *Improving Reading Instruction;*
   Harcourt, Brace & World, Inc., New York, 1956.

O. L. ZANGWILL: "Dyslexia in Relation to Cerebral
   Dominance" in *Reading Disability: Progress and
   Research Needs in Dyslexia;* Johns Hopkins Uni-
   versity Press, Baltimore, 1962.

To My Mother
LOUISE NELSON CROSBY
in fulfillment of
a childhood promise

Contents

Part IV. SUGGESTIONS FOR THERAPY

Introduction

AN EXPLANATION is in order concerning this collaboration in authorship. I am a neurologist and neurosurgeon with a practice exclusively pediatric. According to *Stedman's Medical Dictionary,* a neurologist is "one versed in the science of neurology; a specialist in the treatment of nervous disorders." Neurology is defined as "the branch of medical science that has to do with the nervous system and its disorders." A neurosurgeon is "a surgeon specializing in operations on the nerves and the central nervous system," which includes the brain and the spinal cord. With all due respect to Stedman's, I prefer my own definition. I say a neurologist diagnoses and treats diseases of the nervous system *medically,* while a neurosurgeon diagnoses and treats them *surgically.*

Why restrict practice to children? Because in children a neurologist and/or a neurosurgeon is working with a developing brain. The organic function of the brain is not complete until a person is approximately eighteen years old. In a surgical operation, for example, it is not only necessary to know the immediate effect of the operative procedure, as in an adult, but to estimate its effect in the future. In diagnosing a child's present neurological disorder, it is necessary not only to estimate his present handicap, but his future development as well. Thus I feel that working with children commands full attention.

Mr. Liston is a professional writer. The physician-writer collaboration was arranged because we wanted this book to be as accurate as possible, yet readable by people not trained in medicine. The neurological reading disorders which are the subject of this book cry aloud for a wide audience. For too long, discussion of these disorders has been limited to the medical profession. Parents, teachers, laymen generally need to be informed if a solution to the educational problems posed by these handicapped youngsters is ever to be found.

The road to this collaboration was a bit long. Studies at the University of Chicago in 1952 led to an association with Dr. Douglas N. Buchanan, professor of neurology and pediatrics. Among his interests was *dyslexia,* a neurological disorder of reading. It was here that I was first introduced to this disability and to the subtleties of pediatric neurology.

The University of Chicago was also fortunate to have on its faculty Drs. Helen and Alan Robinson, who have done original and important work in reading disorders. Dr. Joseph Wepman was a member of the medical faculty as well. The University was a major center of reading studies, and Dr. Buchanan worked with the Robinsons in many of their diagnostic problems. Thus it became inevitable that anyone exposed to Dr. Buchanan should become interested in neurological reading disorders.

Upon returning to practice in Baltimore, I encountered a dyslexic patient who was enrolled in the Catholic school system. I contacted the Right Reverend Leo J. McCormick, who was then superintendent of Catholic education, to ask what program he had for dyslexic youngsters. He was not familiar with dyslexia, but he was interested and asked me to contact the director of the Educational and Child Guidance Clinic operated by the school system, Sister Mary Rachel, S.S.N.D. Sister Rachel was unfamiliar with dyslexia also, but asked me to come over and discuss it. Out of that hour's discussion came a most rewarding association. Sister Rachel's clinic saw one hundred or more problem readers a year. When in doubt about the nature of the reading disorders, she asked me to examine the patients. Many, many interesting cases came to me in this way, as they also did from the public-school systems of Baltimore City and surrounding counties. In time, I was asked to talk to teachers and parents' organizations and explanations of dyslexia became involved. There was obviously great need for something laymen could read that would inform them about the problem and answer questions.

Into this situation came Mr. Liston, during the illness of a member of his family. His interest and our mutual conviction of the great need for public exposure to a problem have resulted in this book. The aim of it is to expose an unrecognized problem and to appeal for acceptance that the problem exists. Those who feel that one should not expose a problem without offering a suitable solution may be rather dissatisfied. In the 32 formal case histories we present, such people may find it unsettling that most have a disorder for which little or nothing has been done—but that is precisely the problem we are exposing.

It is customary in the practice of medicine for the physician first to diagnose a disease and then to prescribe treatment. In neurological reading disorders, a physician can diagnose, but he cannot treat. There are no pills to "cure" it, no operative techniques, no exercises to perform. Treatment of the diagnosed disorders lies with the educators and that, too, is part of the reason for this book, to spur teachers to a search for treatment programs for these neurologically impaired youngsters.

Readers may find themselves asking: For whom are they writing? Parents? Teachers? Psychologists? Physicians? We realize it is customary to write for just one of these groups, but in this instance we have endeavored to write for all of them. The point will be made in this book that any solution to the problems of the dyslexic child must include the unique contributions of all four of these groups. There is little point in exposing the problem to parents, for example, when they cannot solve it without the help of teachers, psychologists and physicians.

We have deliberately written for these four groups of specialists—and parents are specialists—for another reason. The problem of the dyslexic child exists unrecognized and unresolved largely because these four specialists have not found a way to talk to each other. Neurologists have known of dyslexia for fifty years or more but have not communicated that knowledge to other medical specialists, let alone psychologists, teachers and parents. This is most regrettable. All of us must find a way to sit down and discuss this educational problem of several million of our youngsters. We cannot continue to waste their talents. This book is an effort to begin discussion.

Our broad approach to reading and dyslexia may create some problems for readers. It is necessary, for example, to provide some background information for parents who lack the expertise of the teacher, psychologist and physician. The latter three groups may find such information somewhat of an oversimplification. We can only ask their indulgence. Similarly, parents who lack technical expertise may find some parts of this to be far from casual reading, but then this is not a simple problem. There is no doubt in our minds that many of our readers, particularly teachers, psychologists and physicians, will want a great deal more information than we have provided, particularly about brain function and neurophysiology. Unfortunately, brain function is so complex that one cannot describe it briefly. Sizable tomes have been devoted to description of the functions of sections of the brain no larger than one's fist, and then have been incomplete. This complexity of the brain has made, virtually without exception, the quasi scientific articles about brain function in the popular press pure, unmitigated drivel.

We have included a great deal of information about brain function, but we have limited it to that which is essential to the understanding of neurological learning disorders. Hopefully, our readers, particularly those with educational and medical expertise, will want to know more. Therefore, we have provided a bibliography suitable for the layman, as well as for the most expert. We have also included annotated notes for those who would like to pursue studies of reading problems.

The organizational plan of this book is rather simple. There are four parts. The first is a general description of dyslexia. Part Two is devoted to normal reading or, more accurately, the manner in which a child without neurological deficiencies learns to read. This material is essential for, unless we first realize how a normal child learns to read, we cannot understand the difficulties of the abnormal child and begin to help him surmount his problems. Part Two may be somewhat controversial. Our views concerning how a normal child learns to read and thereby ought to be taught to read are sometimes in sharp contrast to other opinions and current educational practices. We emphasize that it is not our intention to become involved in a controversy over current methods of reading instruction. We believe the normal child will learn to read no matter how he is taught. But we also believe that many current methods of instruction make learning to read exceedingly difficult for the child with neurological disorders. Part Three is devoted to those disorders, and Part Four contains some suggestions for solutions to the problems of the dyslexic child.

We would like to express our gratitude to those who have directly or indirectly assisted in the preparation of this book:

Dr. Douglas N. Buchanan, who introduced me to dyslexia and taught me what neurology I know.

Dr. James G. Arnold, Professor of Neurosurgery, and Dr. J. Edmund Bradley, Professor of Pediatrics (retired) at the University of Maryland School of Medicine under whom I have worked so happily.

Sister Mary Rachel, and her co-workers, of the Department of Catholic Education, Archdiocese of Baltimore.

Dr. I. H. Weiner and Dr. G. Lee Russo, my associates, and their secretaries, Mrs. Frayda Cohen and Mrs. Evelyn Landau, for their assistance and tolerance.

Mrs. Margaret Cardwell and Miss Pat Donohue, secretaries at Sister Rachel's clinic, for their many kindnesses.

Dr. Raymond Clemmens, Dr. Ray Hepner, Dr. Albert Powell, Mrs. Judith Pazourek, Miss Dorothy G. Sleep for reading the manuscript.

The most helpful staffs of the University of Maryland Health Sciences Library in Baltimore and the McKeldin Library in College Park, Maryland, especially Mrs. Marlene Ances.

Dr. Harry Levin of Cornell University, who gave us a copy of the complete reading-research study which we found so useful.

All my previous secretaries, Mrs. Caroll Hudson Swarm, Mrs. Grace Curtis Petty, Miss Val Hastings, Mrs. Barbara Miller and Mrs. Esther Malin Sherer. But most especially my present secretary, Mrs. Margaret Gill Parsons, who found many of the cases from my meager description, assembled, corrected and typed the manuscript, and performed many other services which are passed over by the usual secretary.

Mr. Philip King of the National Education Association, who supplied useful information.

The wives of the authors, and their children, not only for their encouragement and helpful suggestions, but for their usually willing acceptance of their "book widowhood" and "orphanhood."

All the psychologists with whom I have worked and learned so much, particularly Mike Deem for the many "psychoneurological" bull sessions which were so stimulating.

And above all, my gratitude goes to those patients who taught me so much. I was spurred to write this book by the many encouraging comments from parents and, particularly, from the children themselves, when they learned of the existence and nature of these disorders. But if one person had to be singled out, it would be a retired school teacher who commented following a talk to a school PTA meeting: "Looking back over the many years I taught, I always remember a handful of children I was never able to teach to read. I always felt badly about my failure and wondered whatever became of these youngsters. I only wish I had known then what I have just learned about dyslexia. I might have been able to help them."

Since these words were first published in 1968 there has been an increase in interest and awareness concerning problems of reading disability. Articles and books have appeared. The number of private schools for dyslexic children has increased, but the growth in public school programs has not been proportionate. Where public school programs were started, they were more the result of parental pressure rather than of design within the educational system.

Today, the status of education for children with reading disorders is extremely uneven. One public school may have an enlightened administration and a dedicated and trained staff of remedial reading teachers, while another school has an administration which denies the existence of the problem. It is not uncommon for me to have to tell parents where to move to find a suitable school for their child. We still have a very long way to go in realizing that dyslexia and related disorders are medical problems for which the treatment is educational, and in developing the requisite educational facilities so these many children can take their rightful place in society.

R. M. N. CROSBY, M.D.

Baltimore, Maryland

PART ONE

STATEMENT
OF THE PROBLEM

I.

Introducing Dyslexia

BEING ABLE TO READ is essential in our society. Our whole scheme of learning from "Run, Spot, Run" to an astrophysical analysis of the properties of quasars depends upon the ability to read. A child may have the capacity to write literature, walk upon the surface of the moon or define the true nature of man as he ponders his Maker, but he cannot do any of it unless he first learns to read.

It is true that an illiterate person can become a great painter, a startling inventor of the tinkering variety, a wise and goodly man in his relationship with his fellowman. Such inspiring people exist all over the world. But in our American society, if only because of compulsory education to age sixteen, reading is an absolute essential to happiness and productivity.

There are several reasons that children become problem readers. Some are idle, or lack intelligence, or have emotional problems, or are culturally deprived or were poorly taught. Teachers and school psychologists are accustomed to recognizing and assisting children with such problems.

But there is another major cause for reading difficulties with which teachers and psychologists are far less familiar. Three to four million youngsters have neurological reading disorders, a brain dysfunction which inhibits their ability to learn to read. It is these youngsters, numbering at least ten percent and perhaps as much as fifteen percent of all youngsters entering the first grade, whom we call "the Waysiders."

Though they may be of average or above-average intelligence, they fall behind in their studies, fail grades, develop emotional

3

problems because of frustration, embarrassment and ridicule. Classroom teachers use every means they know to try to teach these children to read well, yet nearly all methods consistently fail. The children remain casualties of education. They fall by the wayside in our rush for education and all the satisfaction and wealth it brings.

In a word, the Waysiders have *dyslexia,* a neurological condition known to medicine for over half a century. Dyslexia and its related disabilities—*dysgraphia,* inability to write, and *dyscalculia,* inability to do arithmetic—can be diagnosed. Although these impairments are not medically treatable, there is no reason why methods of instruction cannot be devised—and some have been—so these children can learn to read at least well enough to obtain sufficient knowledge to make a contribution to society commensurate with their intelligence.

THE NATURE OF DYSLEXIA

Dyslexia is not a disease. Nor is it a syndrome, ailment or infirmity. Dyslexia* is a *symptom* resulting from one or more of various neurological impairments. These causes of dyslexia will be described in great detail in chapters to come, but at this preliminary stage we can say that the symptom known as dyslexia most often appears when a person has impaired visual or auditory perception.

Visual and auditory perception are brain functions which have no relationship to the functions of the eyes and ears. A child may

---

* There is a sizable body of medical literature about dyslexia. This literature shows the authors using several semi-synonymous terms to describe the same condition: word blindness, specific dyslexia, constitutional dyslexia, familial dyslexia, secondary dyslexia, developmental dyslexia, strephosymbolia, congenital symbol-amblyopia, congenital typholexia, specific reading disability, bradylexia, analfabetia partialis, amnesia visualis verbalis, primary reading retardation, and others. To simplify this presentation, we are using the word "dyslexia" to include all organic neurological reading disability.

A number of researchers have attempted to differentiate between *alexia* and *dyslexia,* some insisting that alexia is an acquired condition while dyslexia is congenital. The derivation of the words indicates that dyslexia is a disability and alexia is the total absence of reading ability. When we refer to dyslexia we are not talking about the origin or cause of the complaint or age at onset. We will never refer to alexia, because we have never seen a case of total absence of reading ability.

have 20/20 vision, but if he has visual imperception he fails to distinguish between shapes or patterns. New eyeglasses or larger type will not help his problem. For example, his brain does not perceive the difference between the shape of a triangle and a square. Another child may have the ability to hear the most distant sound or the quietest whisper, but not grasp the difference between the sounds he hears. Thus, he may not recognize that a melody is played in a different key or distinguish the sounds of the short and long *e*.

Human beings can read because they have the neurological ability to recognize the shapes of the individual letters in their alphabet and the words they form and distinguish the sounds those letters and words make. The burden of this book is that a significant percentage of children have an impairment of their neurological ability to perceive shapes and sounds correctly and therefore have reading problems. They are dyslexic.

No one should have the slightest difficulty accepting the fact that such neurological disorders exist. We all understand there are individuals with the capacity to be great artists, blending oils and watercolors into canvases of great beauty and significance. We also understand that there are individuals who are color-blind and thus barred from careers as oil painters, or who simply have a less refined sense of color so that they enjoy fewer of the hues made by man or nature. Other illustrations could be given, but the point is that no one should be the least bit surprised at the existence of people who have great difficulty perceiving the shapes of letters and words and the sounds they represent.

If a person is color-blind or tone-deaf, he is not considered handicapped. His is an inconvenience, perhaps, a brain dysfunction which robs him of some of the esthetic joys of life. But if a person has a brain impairment which inhibits his ability to read, he is robbed of an education, knowledge, meaningful employment, opportunity for a decent standard of living, and most of the satisfaction and higher pleasures of life.

If we pursue further the causes of the symptom known as dyslexia, we will discover that, while the condition may be rooted in poor visual perception or imperfect auditory perception, it most often occurs with one or more of several other minor neurological disorders. Along with his impaired visual perception, a child may have a disorder of tactile perception, that is, he fails to distinguish the shape of an object which he touches. Thus he may not recognize the shapes of coins which he fondles in his pocket. In addition to his visual imperception, he may have an impairment of his ability to perform fine motor skills, that is, coordinate his body so that he can do precise tasks such as tying a knot or walking a straight line. He may have a poor sense of direction and several other neurological discrepancies which we will describe in detail. Along with his reading problem, this dyslexic child may have great difficulty writing, or he may be less than brilliant in arithmetic.

What must be emphasized is that these difficulties are exceedingly minor. Dyslexia is not a gross neurological malady such as polio or "cerebral palsy." The dyslexic child does not usually limp, tremble, wear thick spectacles, have a speech impediment, or seem mentally dull. Rather, he gives every indication of being a normal child. He may be bright and intelligent, personable, athletic, mischievous, everything boys and girls are everywhere—until he goes to school. His is a minimal brain dysfunction, evidenced only in the extremely fine tasks human beings are called upon to do in our complex society. He may be a hard-charging fullback in football, but become disorganized when called upon to perform different tasks with each hand—on the order of the childhood game of patting the head and rubbing the abdomen. While excellent at whitewashing the back fence, he may be less than neat when attempting to draw a circle inside a half-inch square so that it touches all four sides. He may excel at rubbing up a baseball and throwing a curve, but fail to recognize the number 3 when traced on his fingerpads when his eyes are closed.

There are many manifestations of fine neurological function which may (or may not) pose problems for the dyslexic child. The point is that these extremely minor disabilities don't matter and therefore go unnoticed until the child enters school. Then, all of a sudden, he is called upon to distinguish the shapes of letters that really aren't very different, *c* and *o*, for example, *u* and *v*, *w* and *m*, *p* and *q*, *b* and *d*, and many more. These letters are small objects and quite similar. Not only has he to discriminate one from the other, he has to recognize the minute differences between the sounds of a short *a* and a short *i*, for example. He has to learn these letters and the various sounds they represent, then arrange them in very precise ways into words, sentences and paragraphs. Moreover, he is called upon to perform exacting movements with his arm, hand and fingers so as to write these letters, the shapes of which he has difficulty recognizing.

If we are going to recognize, understand and assist these dyslexic children in the fundamentally important task of learning to read, we must discard some preconceived notions. First, these children are not mentally retarded. They are not stupid in any sense of the word. They are intelligent—often extremely intelligent. They can and do learn, by all the methods individuals learn, other than by reading. Many of them partially surmount their reading deficiencies by developing highly-refined oral memories, just as many blind individuals concentrate on their ability to listen.

It may be helpful in understanding these children if we point out that no two people are neurologically the same or that no one is neurologically perfect. We all have eccentricities. We may have a poor sense of direction, or misjudge distances, or find mathematical computation somewhat difficult. We may be less than well coordinated so that we find tennis and golf and swimming more difficult to learn than other individuals. There are an infinite number of individual arrangements of neurological abilities. Our neurological idiosyncrasies are in part what make each of us unique. As we grow up we become acquainted with our abilities and limitations. We plan our life and occupation around them.

The dyslexic child is absolutely no different from the rest of mankind. Unfortunately, his neurological peculiarities happen to make it hard for him to read and write, and it is exceedingly difficult for him to plan his life around these limitations. He poses a most serious educational problem, but he is far from a cripple. Some of us have blue eyes and some of us are left-handed, and others of us have poor visual perception and still others have limited auditory perception. If we can accept blue eyes and left-handedness, we can accept dyslexia.

Another notion that has to go is that dyslexics are "brain-damaged" children. We must discard the idea that these children have a disease of the brain or have sustained a brain injury. There are children who are dyslexic as a result of an accident, illness or some other traumatic occurrence, but these youngsters are a small minority of cases.

What are the causes, then, of the perceptual impairments? For at least half of them, the impairment is genetic in origin. We know, for example, a family of three sisters, all of whom had at least one male child who had a reading disorder. The sisters also had at least one brother who was similarly afflicted. We have traced dyslexia through four generations of another family, as in Illustration 1.

Dyslexia does not always follow this genetic pattern. Reading disorders may strike both male and female members of a family. In a family of six children, several of whom are patients, the oldest son is now an honor student in high school, but had remedial-reading instruction in the third grade; the next son, two years younger, has had a great deal of remedial-reading instruction; the third son, again two years younger, is eight and a half years old and reads at the first-grade level; the fourth child, a girl, was seen in a suburban school system and diagnosed as dyslexic; a fourth boy has had remedial reading; and the second girl, six and a half, can't write the alphabet. She left out the *u* and *v*, explaining that she "couldn't remember what they looked like."

Or, dyslexia may affect only certain members of a family. Among a family of seven children, the two oldest have no learning disabilities, but the remaining five all have reading problems. Each successive sibling has a greater disability. The youngest, seven and a half and a very bright child, cannot identify most of the letters of the alphabet. When shown a letter on a flashcard, he said, "Oh, yes, that's the one with the dirt on it. That's a *j*."

Such familial instances of dyslexia are so striking that it has led some observers to exaggerate the congenital nature of dyslexia. While dyslexia and other neurological learning disorders do "run in families," we believe this accounts for approximately half the cases. We have seen an equal number of cases in which there is no family history of reading disorders. Only an isolated child is affected.

This observation, which others have made, too, leads to the conclusion that neurological reading disorders can be both genetic in origin and acquired.

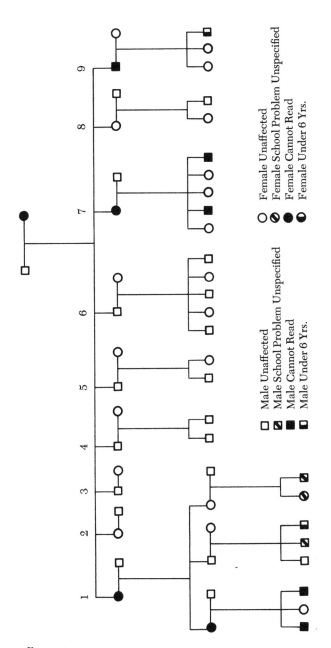

Illustration 1

How is it acquired? Readers may find this answer unsatisfactory, but, barring serious head injury or other such extremes, it is only possible to say that definite causes are unknown. It is likely that many of the children, quite early in infancy, may have undergone minimal brain dysfunction which was unobserved by parents and physician, but that explanation does not reveal much to parents or patients. What is important at this point is to realize the impairment is quite minor and that it exists. For those who are dyslexic and for their parents and teachers, the central problem is to surmount the resulting educational difficulties.

If we are to understand dyslexia, we must realize it is not a case of measles. A physician does not diagnose on the basis of a fever, a sore throat and a skin rash, put the patient to bed and prescribe some medication. There are no pills, no "shots," no surgical techniques to "cure" dyslexia. For the neurologist, the frustrating aspect of his work with dyslexia is that he can diagnose, but he cannot treat. Therapy is largely the realm of the educator.

Another preconceived notion to be eliminated if we are to understand dyslexia is the conception of the brain as a series of "little black boxes," each controlling some body function. There are a few body functions which can be localized in some area of the brain, but reading and writing involve such an array of brain function that almost the entirety of the brain is encompassed. There are no "damaged" areas to be pointed to as the "cause" of the reading disorder. We are dealing here with a brain function that is amorphous and ambiguous.

In examining the nature of dyslexia, we can say that it occurs three to four times as frequently among males as females. A number of reasons have been offered for this, including the somewhat slower maturation of males. None of the reasons advanced seems to offer a satisfactory explanation, so at present we can only say that no one knows why neurological learning disorders affect males more often.

Another characteristic of such reading disorders is that they may be permanent or transient. A child may have impaired visual perception, for example, and bear the disability all his life. Or—and we believe it is the more common occurrence—the impairment may exist only in childhood and improve, sometimes disappearing, with age. We have seen many cases wherein the child had a disorder which affected his learning in the primary grades, but showed remarkable improvement as he approached his teens.

Any discussion of the nature of dyslexia must take cognizance of its relationship to handedness. The simple fact that dyslexia occurs more often among left-handed people than right-handed has both confused and enamored those few educators who have investigated dyslexia. The problem of left-right dominance will be a subject of a subsequent chapter, but at this preliminary stage it is necessary only to state that there is a relationship between dyslexia and handedness, albeit a confused one.

One more characteristic of dyslexia must be cited. Each dyslexic child is unique. He may have a simple disorder unaccompanied by other neurological difficulties, or he may have a complex array of neurological peculiarities. Indeed, to the consternation of those who observe the phenomenon, a patient may have no *demonstrable* perceptual or motor difficulties, yet still have dyslexia! The variegated nature of dyslexia is its greatest challenge to parents, educators and physicians. Each child must be separately diagnosed and a plan of therapy must be developed which fits the unique problems of each child. Some educational grouping of dyslexics may be possible, but in the main we are dealing with the staggering problem of providing essentially individual tutoring for millions of youngsters. A child may have difficulty reading and that difficulty may be based in his inability to perceive the shapes of letters and words or in his failure to recognize the sounds they represent—or both—or it may have some other neurological cause. He may have difficulty in both reading and writing, in writing but not reading. He may have a problem in arithmetic as well as reading and writing, or in arithmetic and reading, or in arithmetic and writing. And he may have any of these conditions from a mild to a severe degree, and his condition may improve with the passage of time or it may not.

THE PLIGHT OF THE DYSLEXIC CHILD

That so many millions of youngsters are taught to read every year is the mark of the genius and persistence of teachers and the diligence of their often reluctant pupils, many of whom would rather play baseball. A far greater number and much larger percentage of children are learning to read now than ever before in our history. Our teachers have tried *everything* they know and can think of to teach the Waysiders to read. As Charles G. Fries, emeritus professor of English at the University of Michigan, has so eloquently put it: "If 'Johnny can't read,' it is not because his teachers, or the principal of his school, or the superintendent of his school system, or the professors of education, or the psychologists, or the directors of reading clinics, have ignored or neglected the problems created by the innumerable and diverse Johnnies and Janes that must, for modern living, have an increasingly high standard of literacy. Whatever the causes of the 'failure of modern education,' no one can insist that they have arisen out of willful neglect of the problems or an unwillingness to labor hard in their study."[1]* Nor have the efforts been in vain. American education has sharply reduced the percentage of problem readers.

Yet the fact remains that our educational system, while geared to help all handicapped children, ignores the dyslexic child. If a child is mentally retarded, he is enrolled in special classes, graded in relation to his ability, where he is taught those skills which he is able to learn. If a child is physically handicapped so that he is confined to crutches, braces or a wheelchair, he is transported to schoolrooms where less physical movement is required. If he is deaf, he is enrolled in classes equipped to make the most of his limited hearing and to teach him to speak. If he has impaired vision, he is enrolled in sight-saving classes where he uses large type and other devices to make full use of his sight; or if he is totally blind, he attends classes where he learns Braille. If he has a brain disorder which causes him to be aphasic, he is dispatched to special schools where an effort is made to help him understand and speak his native language. But if a child is dyslexic, with very few exceptions, no special classes exist for him. True, he attends remedial-reading classes, but these are often geared to reteach by the same methods that have already failed. Except for a few fortunate individuals, the dyslexic child does not receive the benefit of a precise diagnosis and careful plan of individualized instruction, as other handicapped youngsters do.

---

* Numbered notes will be found in the Bibliographical Notes section at the end of the book.

Consider the plight of this youngster. As will be shown in detail, reading is the most complex and difficult neurological assignment a person is called upon to perform in his lifetime, exceeding in difficulty even the involved task of learning to speak. It is more than pertinent that the child is granted years in which to learn to speak, but only months in which to learn to read and write. And, though the hickory stick has long vanished from the classroom, learning to read and write is done in an essentially punitive atmosphere: if the child fails or even just has difficulty learning, he will be installed in a slow group, fail the grade, disappoint his parents and incur the ridicule of his classmates. For six and a half years he has been the apple of his parents' eyes, a great baseball player, an expert fisherman, a superior teller of tall tales, confident he can lick the world. Now he finds himself a failure at the important task of reading. He does not understand why all his effort and determination do not help him, and he is far more disappointed even than his parents or teachers.

Almost everything that happens to him thereafter compounds his problem. He is sent to school psychologists, social workers, nurses and doctors. He is probed, prodded, tested, questioned, talked to and admonished, if not parentally deprived of privileges and corporally punished. He enters remedial-reading classes—and, as is far from exceptional, is even relegated to classes for retarded children. If the child rebels or withdraws from this process and comes to hate himself and dislike school, teachers, parents and all the others who are bothering but not helping him, who is to blame him? If he decides to compensate for his scholastic failure by succeeding at mischief, misbehavior, or even delinquency, who can fail to understand it?

RECOGNIZING THE DYSLEXIC CHILD

We do not blame educators for failing to recognize and help the dyslexic child in the special ways in which he needs help. Dyslexia is so very minor. Except in school or when called upon to read, the dyslexic can perform well. Nor is he a total failure even in school. He learns in all the ways one learns other than by reading, orally from what the teacher and other students say and from movies, television and other visual aids. He even learns to read—some. We have seen some very severe cases of dyslexia, but we have never seen a child who cannot learn to read at least a few words. The problem of the dyslexic child is that he does not read up to standard.

The teacher has difficulty recognizing the dyslexic child because he often looks like all the other slow readers she is accustomed to helping. He may appear to be either lazy, mentally slow, culturally deprived or emotionally disturbed, and, in a way, he is all these things, but for different reasons. Particularly in the upper elementary grades, he may become lazy because of his discouragement over his reading. He is intellectually retarded and culturally deprived because he has read less and therefore knows less. He may be a behavioral problem and may have emotional disorders that stem from his frustration about reading. The point is that all of these symptoms of a poor reader who is not dyslexic also result from a child's failure to read due to a neurological disability.

Nearly every teacher has encountered the dyslexic child and not realized what he has seen. No better illustration of this exists than in John Holt's poignant book, *How Children Fail.*[2] Holt has taught English, French and math in elementary and junior-high schools, and has done educational research in several private schools. As demonstrated in his book, he has deep understanding and empathy for children—such as Emily, whom he described in this passage:

> Remember when Emily, asked to spell "microscopic," wrote "mincopert"? That must have been several weeks ago. Today I wrote "mincopert" on the board. To my great surprise, she recognized it. Some of the kids, watching me write it, said in amazement, "What's that for?" I said, "What do you think?" Emily answered, "It's supposed to be 'microscopic.'" But she gave not the least sign of knowing that she was the person who had written 'mincopert.' "
>
> On the diagnostic spelling test, she spelled "tariff" as "tearerfit." Today I thought I would try her again on it. This time she wrote "tearfit." What does she do in such cases? Her reading aloud gives a clue. She closes her eyes and makes a dash for it, like someone running past a graveyard on a dark night. No looking back afterward, either. . . .

Is this the way some of these children make their way through life?

Then Holt continues with a "Memo to the Research Committee" as follows: "I have mentioned Emily, who spelled 'microscopic' as 'mincopert.' She obviously made a wild grab at an answer, and having written it down, never looked at it, never checked to see if it looked right. I see a lot of this one-way, don't-look-back-it's-too-awful strategy among students."

At this writing, we have never met Holt, nor have we ever had occasion to meet Emily. But based solely on Holt's description, there is a definite indication that Emily has a rather severe dyslexia and dysgraphia. One can only hope that Holt's curiosity about this child led him to suggest a neurological examination so that the precise nature of her dyslexia and dysgraphia could be determined. In any event, Holt has given an excellent description of the performance of a dyslexic child in a classroom setting, and indicated the concern teachers have over these children.

The solution in such cases is to have a careful psychological and neurological examination made to determine the nature of brain dysfunction and permit teachers to plan an instructional program. We are not suggesting routine neurological examinations for all children. We will, however, point out some peculiarities of these dysfunctions which may be clues to parents and teachers that the basis of the child's reading problem may be neurological. A visit to the neurologist at that time would be most wise.

EDUCATION PROBLEMS

In this brief introduction to dyslexia, we have tried to summarize the nature of the disorders, the plight of the child and the problem the teacher has in recognizing him. In so doing, we have endeavored to show that dyslexia is unlike the illnesses which we are accustomed to our children having, that it is a strange disorder occurring rather commonly and that it has many, many forms so that it poses a considerable problem in diagnosis and a Gargantuan task for the educators who must teach dyslexics to read and write.

We are not suggesting that the educational problems are hopeless. These children can be taught to read, if not well, at least sufficiently to make use of their abilities and lead a productive life. But the Waysiders cannot always be taught by some present methods of instruction. The whole-word or look-say method of instruction is a disaster for the child with impaired visual perception. Similarly, the phonic approach is less than productive for the child with auditory imperception. Nor will the kinesthetic method work for the child who has poor tactile perception.

Yet we believe there are methods which will work. We will suggest what some methods might be, but we insist we are not educators, psychologists, remedial-reading instructors or preparers of basal readers and textbooks. We are only exposing a problem. The real therapeutic solutions to these problems must be developed by the educators working in cooperation with psychologists, physicians and parents.

But before we can begin to develop techniques to teach dyslexic children, we must first examine present methods of instruction to see how they fail to meet the needs of the dyslexic child and, in fact, often intensify his problem.

2.

The Missing Ingredient

THE CURRENT EDITION of the authoritative *Subject Guide to Books in Print (U.S.A.)* lists 841 titles on the subject of reading. This total does not include readers, that is, books used by pupils in learning to read. Nor does it encompass volumes on literature, history, geography or any other subject taught in school.

These are 841 books on the art and science of reading, with titles ranging from *Operation Alphabet* and *Free to Read* to *The Relation of Certain Anomalies of Vision and Lateral Dominance to Reading Disability.* In short, these are books written by various experts stating their views on how reading can be taught to non-readers and how this delicate art can be improved in poor readers.

These 841 books are only a small part of the total medical and scientific literature on the subject. One study[1]—a sort of study of studies—maintains there are "more than 20,000 articles and books devoted to reading retardation."

Too little space in these books and articles is devoted to dyslexia and other neurological learning disorders. Those writings by educators which do mention dyslexia treat it as a rare phenomenon which the average teacher would not be expected to encounter in her lifetime. Seldom if ever do these educators indicate any awareness that present methods of reading instruction might be less than helpful to the dyslexic child or that they might worsen his problem.

THE EXTENT OF THE READING PROBLEM

How many children are problem readers—that is, read two years or more below their grade level or, if they read at grade level, do it so slowly they cannot keep pace informationally with their classmates? No census has ever been taken nor does it seem possible that one could be. In lieu of one, scholars and educators have estimated the reading problem. Our study of these estimates shows they range from a low of ten percent to a high of 75 percent.[2] Those who have studied dyslexia estimate that ten percent to 25 percent of all beginning readers are affected.

We have no desire to overstate the problem. It is bad enough in any event. We are saying that ten percent of all elementary children have a reading problem rooted in neurological disorders. They are the Waysiders, the hard core of problem readers who exist year in and year out despite the intense labor of their teachers. Not all, fortunately, are severe cases. A sizable majority have a mild to moderate dyslexia that is transient in nature, but every one of these three to four million youngsters is a potential reading problem if he is not given special attention.

In recent years many studies have been made of the fate of the problem reader. These studies show that he wastes his potential, drops out of school, develops emotional problems, becomes delinquent. He is unemployed and often unemployable, a victim of poverty and a drain on society. There are many exceptions, of course, but in the main, the problem reader remains a major and most difficult social and economic problem.[3]

The reading problem is worsening despite the diligent efforts of educators. Since our technological age places greater emphasis on scholarship and higher education, the informational lag of the problem reader is greater. The poor reader of today is intellectually, culturally and economically worse off than his slow-reading grandfather.[4]

METHODS OF TEACHING READING ARE UNCHANGED

The 20,000 articles and books devoted to the immense and seemingly unsolvable reading problem show that some rather prominent people feel that modern educational research has greatly revised our methods of reading instruction. A case in point is an article by Dr. Nila Banton Smith entitled "Trends in Beginning Reading Since 1900." This appears in *Teaching Young Children to Read,* the premier brochure of the United States Office of Education. It has been distributed by the millions by the Government Printing Office.

In her article, Dr. Smith states that the era beginning in 1920 brought "revolutionary changes in attitudes toward teaching reading to beginners and drastic revisions in school practices." She states that by 1900, the alphabetic approach to reading, that is, teaching a child the letters and having him memorize the arrangement of them in a word, had all but disappeared in the United States. The phonic approach to reading, which she says began in the 1890s, was in full swing. After 1920, reading readiness became a vogue and "oral reading was abandoned, and the concept of teaching silent reading burst into our slumbering complacency like a bombshell." Reading tests were developed, a necessity under silent reading, and school administrators "were shocked to find that thousands of children could not read and that most of the ones who could read knew little of what they were reading."

Dr. Smith says the "whole problem was blamed on the strong emphasis that had been placed upon what the educators of the time called 'juggling with meaningless phonic elements.' And so, phonics was practically abandoned, and reading methods swung to the other extreme of an exaggerated emphasis on silent reading for meaning."

The twenties and thirties brought an Activity Movement, with children working "freely and spontaneously and actively in following their own interests." Classrooms were filled with children hammering and cooking and painting and sewing and modeling. "Experience materials for reading now became a strong trend."

The 1940s and war brought more emphasis on systematized reading programs and "almost universal use of basal readers." The Armed Forces charged that too many American young men could not read (just as today!). This was followed by a return to grace of phonics. This method of reading was found, after study, to have merit after all. "Phonics was now reinstated with renewed confidence," writes Dr. Smith, "but with a different timing, in a different method, and in combination with other word-attack approaches. Findings in regard to timing are pertinent insofar as teaching reading to young children is concerned. Two studies had indicated that children could not make the best use of formal phonics instruction until they had arrived at a mental age of seven years. In the light of these studies, phonics was generally delayed until the second grade."

Commenting on trends since 1950, Dr. Smith finds the major influence on reading is "public pressure resulting from the atomic age," pressure to "produce more competency in a shorter time." She decries the "severe criticism of present methods which are being hurled by laymen and by professional people in other fields." She says, "Many of these critics are either *un*informed or *mis*informed concerning the history of reading and the results of reading research. Their chief contention is that we should return to the type of phonic instruction which was in use from 1900 to 1920."

Dr. Smith points out most emphatically that most of the "new" methods of reading being suggested—"there are phonic methods galore, and we hear of the television method, programmed instruction, the linguistic approach, the individualized plan, the use of the Augmented Roman Alphabet, and so on"—are not new, but rather quite old. "What I am trying to say is that we are not putting new wine in old bottles. We are putting old wine in new bottles. The substance is the same; the container is new."

Another scholar, Dr. Fries, whom we have previously quoted,[5] would agree with Dr. Smith that most of the "new" methods being urged today are quite old. He disagrees most strongly, however, with her view of history. He finds the methods are very, very old. Quoting Dr. Smith, he scores educational research of the last 40 years as having had "comparatively little effect" in developing new methods of teaching.

Professor Fries' view of the history of reading instruction is that most of the theories used today were developed prior to the twentieth century. John Hart, the Englishman, urged a phonic system in the middle 1500s, and he had a clear understanding of the importance of meaning in reading. Many other writers, particularly in the nineteenth century, eloquently described the importance of meaning.

The word or look-say method was fully developed, according

to Professor Fries, in the first half of the nineteenth century. In 1842, *The Common School Journal IV* criticized phonics as "those cadaverous particles, *ba, be, bi, bo, bu*, etc." and denounced "the stiff perpendicular row of characters, lank, stark, immovable, without form or comliness, and as to signification, wholly void." Professor Fries presents in *Linguistics and Reading* a long quote from *The Common School Journal* showing that an individual, in a letter signed simply "M," set out most lucidly the theory and practice of the word method in use today.

One suspects the "M" was Horace Mann, generally considered the "father" of the look-say method. Writing in 1837, Mann criticized phonics as "often a barren action of the organs of speech upon the atmosphere" and suggested that 11/12ths of all children in reading classes did not understand the meanings of the words they read.

Perhaps Mann's most famous statement was this:

> In speaking the word apple, for instance, young children think no more of the Roman letters which spell it than in eating the fruit they think of the chemical ingredients which compose it, hence, presenting them with the alphabet is giving them what they never saw, heard or thought of before. It is as new as algebra and to the eye, not very unlike it, but printed names of known things are the signs of sounds which their ears have become accustomed to hear and their organs of speech to utter and which may excite agreeable feelings and associations. When put to learning the names of the alphabet first, the child has no acquaintance with them, but if put to learning familiar words first, he already knows them by ear, the tongue, and the mind, while his eyes are only unacquainted with them. It can hardly be doubted, therefore, that a child would learn to name twenty-six familiar words much sooner than the unknown, unheard, and unthought-of letters of the alphabet.[6]

Professor Fries reveals in detail that the sentence method and silent reading for meaning were fully developed as theories and practices in the 1870s, then writes: "I have not been able to find the evidence to justify the assertion that the published findings of recent educational research (since 1916) have provided the basis of most of the modern reforms in reading instruction."

This disagreement between two such eminent scholars as Dr. Smith and Professor Fries is not solely an academic one. If

Professor Fries is correct, as we believe he is, then the methods by which children are being taught to read have been basically unchanged in 40 years and perhaps longer. True, there have been improvements and refinements. The books, vocabulary, type size, illustrations have changed. The material is more understandable and meaningful to a young child. The teachers are better trained and equipped with manuals that are very precise in instructing how to teach a child to read. But the methods, despite all the research, are essentially the same old questionable procedures.

> As a matter of fact, [says Professor Fries][7] the educational research of the last forty years seems to have had comparatively little effect in originating new approaches to the teaching of reading. That research studies from 1916 to 1960 (or what some people have believed these research studies had 'proved') may have, from time to time, supported particular practices of certain teachers, or may have contributed to practical decisions concerning materials and methods cannot be denied; but the important changes in approach that characterize the history of the teaching of reading in the schools have grown out of the earnest struggle of the teachers and the administrators themselves to find better ways —ways to achieve specific types of ability that the approach then in use neglected, ways to make their teaching measure up to their ideals of all that must be accomplished.

Professor Fries is clearly unimpressed with modern scientific investigations into the reading problem. He writes:

> One comes away from a concentrated study of hundreds out of the thousands of these investigations much distressed. He seeks in vain for the cumulative continuity that has characterized all recognized sound scientific research. He struggles hard, without success, to find the strands of fundamental assumptions and accepted criteria of sound procedure running through a series of studies attacking any of the major problems of the teaching of reading.

W. S. Gray said:

> Unfortunately, much of the scientific work relating to reading has been fragmentary in character. As pointed out by various writers the investigator frequently attacks an isolated problem, completes his study of it, and suggests that he will continue his research at some later time, but often fails to do so. In the second place, there is far too little coordination of effort among research

workers in the field of reading. . . . In the third place, many of the studies reported have been conducted without adequate controls.[8]

Our point is that educational research in the modern era has not produced any basic improvement over the methods which have failed to eradicate the hard core of problem readers. This educational research most certainly has not taken cognizance of the problems of the dyslexic child.

HOW READING IS TAUGHT TODAY

The noneducator delving into the voluminous educational literature cannot help but be astonished at the controversy that has been carried on over the years about the relative merits of phonics versus the whole word or look-say methods of teaching reading.

The phonic people say that the look-say method is slow and time-consuming. A child who has a speaking vocabulary of 10,000 words when he enters the first grade (some children have twice that) goes to school for nine months and is able to recognize only 300 words by the end of the first grade, having read each one hundreds of times. Worse, knowing these simple words does not help him learn to attack and recognize words that he has never seen, but the meaning of which he knows.

The phonic approach, its advocates maintain, provides the child with the raw materials for reading. The child learns the sounds of the letters and syllables and can use them to pronounce and recognize any word he ever sees.

The reply of the look-sayers is that phonics is quite boring and frustrating and confusing to the child. It stultifies the first-grader's eagerness to read, because he spends such a long time learning sounds and letters and doesn't read. Moreover, many children have great difficulty with phonics and never catch on. Too, there are so many exceptions to "phonic rules" that a child needs considerable maturity to accept the complicated system, they say. Finally, it is argued, phonics was the dominant system for decades and was abandoned simply because of its own demonstrated shortcomings.

In the last half decade, the advocates of phonics and look-say have sought an accommodation. Each has admitted the other method has some advantage. The goal today is an amalgamation of both methods. The result is an infinite variety of methods of teaching reading. Here in Baltimore, the Catholic school system uses virtually a pure phonic method, while many of the surburban Baltimore County public schools use an almost pure look-say method. Phonics is used only in the remedial-reading program. In between these extremes is a variety of combinations of both phonics and look-say. Some have a lot of phonics and others a little with the system varying from school to school, classroom to classroom and even pupil to pupil.

The search for improved ways to use phonics and look-say in the classroom has led to some new developments. One of the most interesting is the Initial Teaching Alphabet (ITA) of 44 characters.[9] This consists of 24 standard, lower-case roman letters (omitting the *q* and *x*) plus 20 additional characters. Each character has only one lower-case form, thus eliminating the child's confusion about capital, lower-case and italicized letters. In addition, each letter has only one sound, thus eliminating approximately 2,000 confusing phonic irregularities. For example, in traditional spelling the *i* sound is different in *child, buy, eye, file, lie, high, aisle, island, guide,* to name a few. The ITA alphabet eliminates this confusion and makes reading much more logical for the child. Later the pupil makes the transition to the regular alphabet.

An example of material written in the new alphabet follows:

ᴄhicken-licken

Wun dæ ᴄhicken-licken

went too ᴛhe wᴑods for fᴑod.

Whiel ʃhee wos ᴛhær an æcorn

fell on her poor littl hed.

"œ! œ!" sed ᴄhicken-licken.

"ᴛhe skie fell on mie hed.

ie must gœ and tell ᴛhe kiŋ."

Professor Fries is an advocate of a linguistics approach to reading. The science of linguistics is an old one but only recently has it been applied to the teaching of reading. The child is taught the alphabet and individual words through their spelling patterns, then is taught to make independent "extensions" of matrices or words that form the basis of hundreds of words in English. Adding prefixes and suffixes to words can rapidly extend a child's reading vocabulary.

These two ways of implementing phonics and look-say, and there are others, are the most highly regarded of the ones developed in recent years. Each has its advocates and is being tried experimentally. The fact remains that most children are taught to read by some variety of the phonic or look-say method. The techniques of their use have changed, but the basic methods are the same that have been in use for many decades.

CLASSROOM INSTRUCTION

The phonic and look-say methods are applied to the schoolroom situation in three principal ways, by far the most common of which is the *Basal Reading Program*. The teacher has a series of basal readers, put out by one of scores of publishing houses, which include books, starting with reading-readiness material and including two to four preprimers, one or two primers, and one or two first readers. There is a set of manuals for the teacher, telling him how to use the books, workbooks tied in with the readers, large word and phrase cards, a "big book" which introduces preprimer reading, and perhaps filmstrips, related storybooks and other books on arithmetic, social studies, health and science.

These basal readers, which the teacher uses in order, are customarily of the look-say type. Dr. Albert J. Harris has determined that the readers, depending on the series in use, endeavor to introduce a first-grader to between 235 to 477 words. He learns these by pure repetition—"Run, Spot, Run"—or in the Ginn Basic Readers:[10]

> Come, Flip.
> Come and see the toys.
> Come and see Susan.
> Come and see Bunny.

In that one page, mostly filled with a large drawing in color, the child has read "come" four times, "and" three times and "see" three times. This goes on for page after page. Professor Charles Walcutt has noted[11] that in the first three grades, a child using the Macmillan series of basal readers learns 1,342 words by repeating them 28,000 times. These readers, staunchly defended by their authors, publishers and school administrators, have been acidly criticized as a vast intellectual wasteland, likely to quench forever a child's interest in reading. We are not about to enter this fray, not so much from lack of courage (but that, too), as from a desire to save our battles for the ones we consider more important.

Teachers habitually add phonics to the basal reading program, in amounts varying from child to child and school system to school system. The phonics is used to enable children to understand and attack words far beyond the limitations of their basal readers. Thus, the child receives the fun and stimulation of learning to read words and "stories" right from the start, while receiving "nuts and bolts" training that will eventually extend his reading horizons.

A second but far less common method of teaching reading is *Language Experience Approach*. In this the teacher endeavors to introduce reading into a total experience setting which includes speaking, listening and writing. The children participate in an interesting experience. Under the guidance of the teacher, they discuss the experience, formulate a title and compose a series of sentences describing their experience. They watch as the teacher writes the group composition on the blackboard and listen as she reads it to them. The story is used for reading instruction of both the look-say and phonics methods.

Thus, a class may have gone to the zoo. A composition is written about the experience, referring to the animals at the zoo, the members of the family who went, the popcorn eaten, etc. The teacher will take a word, *zoo,* for example, and teach it to the children by the look-say method. She may instruct them in the phonics of it and use it in a sentence. Any such experience can be used—a birthday, trip to the firehouse, plants growing in the classroom. Under a capable teacher, this system can be most stimulating to children.

A third method is the *Individualized Approach,* which, en-deavors to group together children with similar reading problems and teach each group differently in accordance with its needs. Each group goes at its own pace using materials that seem most suitable. Each group may receive more emphasis on phonics or less as the teacher judges its need.

Then there is the so-called *Newcastle Experiment* of Dr. Glenn McCracken in Newcastle, Pennsylvania. He enthusiastically supports the use of filmstrips to accompany a basal reading series. Each frame of film shows a colored picture and under it some lines of reading which appear also in the reader. The projected sentences are read aloud, words singled out, pronounced, and analyzed phonetically. Later the children read these words in their reader. Dr. McCracken claims to have obtained excellent results with his system.

Each of these systems, regrettably described so briefly, which do work with some children, has its army of advocates, many of whom feel their system is the cure-all for the nation's reading problem. If properly adopted nationwide, the advocates say, their system would markedly reduce if not eliminate the hard core of problem readers. The trouble is they haven't.

The outpouring of literature about reading shows the educators are quite aware that the methods of instruction heretofore used have not eliminated all of the problem readers. What then are the causes of poor reading? The search for answers has led, inevitably, to the discovery of many causes which range from sound concepts to the purest drivel.

In the main, teachers have concentrated upon four principal causes of reading disorders. First, mental retardation. An observable number of children lack the intellectual capacity to read at the level of the child with average or above-average intelligence. Second, cultural deprivation. The child, particularly from the slums, who grows up in a culturally impoverished environment may be a poor reader. If he has never seen or heard of a cow or a tree or a book, the word will have no meaning for him when he learns to read it. Instead of an oral vocabulary of 10,000 words, which is normal for the first-grader, he may be limited to 2,500 words or less. Correction of this cultural deprivation is the object of Operation Headstart.

The third source of reading disorders of which educators are most conscious is emotional disorders. The child is distracted by worries. Perhaps his is a broken home, or a parent is an alcoholic or ill, or he doesn't get enough to eat, or some other concern interferes with his concentration upon reading. The child may be immature so that he lacks the capacity for study. Or he may have emotional problems stemming from his environment which cripple his motivation and inhibit the learning process. We do not deny that emotional problems are a factor in poor reading, but it is a cause easily overemphasized. One of the origins of a child's emotional problems may simply be that he is a poor reader for neurological reasons. He fails in reading for reasons which he cannot help and which his parents and teachers fail to recognize, and he reacts emotionally.

The fourth cause for reading disorders is lack of adequate teaching. The child may have had inept teachers or he may have been absent from school because of illness or he may have moved to school systems with different methods of instruction.

MYTHS ABOUT THE READING PROBLEM

Along with these legitimate causes of the reading problem have come a number of less than valid reasons. The first is eyesight. It is natural to assume that when a child is a poor reader perhaps he cannot see—to blame the eyes for his failure to read. The eyes are not at fault. True, if a child's visual acuity is less than 20/20, correction should be made, if possible. He should be examined by an ophthalmologist or optometrist and corrective lenses prescribed. Routine administration of the Massachusetts Eye Test in schools is certainly to be encouraged.* Too, if the child's visual acuity is not fully correctable, this fact should be considered in his placement in the classroom. It may be necessary to enroll him in a sight-saving class where large type and other devices are used to aid the child.

But visual acuity has nothing to do with whether or not a child can learn to read. He may have to use large type or Braille, but eyesight has nothing to do with the learning process. There is, in fact, no eye defect which prevents a child from reading. A one-eyed child can read. A child with a "cross-eyed" or "wall-eyed" squint can read. Children with only limited eyesight can read, if only large type. Blind children can learn to read Braille. A child with double vision can learn to read, because he discards one of the images he sees.

Regrettably, many parents of children with eye defects have spent lavishly of their time and substance (not to mention the child's patience) on eye exercises that allegedly will help the child read better. If a child has an eye-muscle imbalance that

---

* Ophthalmologists have begun urging eye examinations for preschoolers in an effort to prevent an eye disorder known as *amblyopia ex anopsia*. If a young child has a refractile difficulty in one eye, he will often discard the image from that eye. If the condition is not discovered and corrected, the child will, usually by age five, irrecoverably lose the vision of the impaired eye. At this writing, ophthalmologists, in conjunction with pediatricians, are planning a national campaign to alert parents to the danger and the need for early examination.

leads to problems in eye convergence, the exercises prescribed may have cosmetic value in correcting these conditions, but they will not be an iota of benefit in helping him to read. The activity might be compared to having a blind child do finger exercises in hope of helping him learn Braille.

A related myth, fortunately receding as a fad, is that faulty eye motions are the root of reading difficulties. As we have seen, we read with the brain, not with the eyes. Thirty years ago or more observers noticed that poor readers had eye movements different from those of experienced readers. In the latter, the eye scans a line making one or more stops, at which time the eye fixes on one or more words. Inexperienced readers and particularly poor readers have eye movements that are irregular. There are frequent stops and reversals as the eye goes back over what has been read.

The production of at least a small papermaking factory has been devoted to a great mass of material analyzing eye movements in reading. This writing may have value to some, but the problem reader is not among them. The problem reader's eye movements are not the cause of his difficulty, but the result. His eye movements are irregular because he reads poorly, studying letters and words individually and reversing himself in an effort to figure out the context.

We are hardly unique in pointing out the lack of significance between eye defects and reading problems. Most of the world's leading neurologists, ophthalmologists and authorities on dyslexia have made similar observations.

Dr. Herman K. Goldberg, Assistant Professor of Ophthalmology at Wilmer Eye Institute, Johns Hopkins Hospital, Baltimore, has said that "far too much emphasis is placed on the importance of good vision as it affects children with reading problems."[12] He said it is wrong to blame faulty eye movement for poor reading. "The converse is actually true. The faulty eye movements are due to poor understanding of the printed words," basing his statement on a study of good and poor readers using an oculonystagmograph to chart the movement of the eyes.

Perhaps the last word should come from Dr. Macdonald Crichley, who is considered the world's leading authority on dyslexia. He said of the eye-motion discussion, "Arguments of this kind are surely topsy-turvy. Faulty eye movements must be regarded as the outcome of a difficulty in reading, and not its cause."[13]

Another myth, or series of myths, relates to medical causes for reading problems. As early as 1922, W. S. Gray listed malnutrition as the cause of reading problems in four children.[14] Willard Olson of the University of Michigan listed hypothyroidism, delay in descent of testicles and similar growth retardation as causes.[15] Donald D. Durrell of Boston University in one of his early writings listed low vitality due to malnutrition, internal glandular disturbances, chorea (St. Vitus Dance), rheumatic fever and low metabolism as factors in reading disorders.[16]

It is significant that these ideas appeared in the early writings of these men. Because these are scholarly men who made many contributions to the study of reading disorders, these less than noteworthy concepts have been repeated by writer after writer in book upon book. Reading has nothing to do with the testicles, other glands, the joints, the heart, liver, bowels or diet. It is past time for this well-meant but erroneous clutter to be removed from the literature on reading disorders.

READING IS A FUNCTION OF THE BRAIN

Many of those who have searched for causes for reading disorders and the best methods to teach reading have neglected an elemental fact: reading is a function of the brain. It is not a function of the eye, for a blind child can learn to read. It is not a function of the ear, for the deaf child can be taught, too. Reading is a brain function, an elemental neurological process in a direct continuum of rolling over, reaching and grasping, sitting, standing, walking, climbing stairs, running, talking, and training bowels and bladder.

Isn't everything a person learns or does a brain function? Of course, but different functions. Geography, history, science, grammar, philosophy, electronics, astrogeology and almost all the other subjects involve the child's *comprehension,* which is one of the functions of the brain. Forward rolls, flips, tumbling, basketball, baseball and other physical accomplishments taught and learned in school are improvements in his basic neurological motor skills developed very early in his life. The physical-education teacher does not instruct the normal child in rolling over, reaching and grasping, walking and running. He learned these before he came to school.

With one exception, the only basic neurological functions taught in school are reading and writing. The exception is arithmetic. There is evidence that calculation is performed in the cortex of the brain. If the child has a dysfunction of this cortical area, he will have difficulty learning arithmetic. He will have a *dyscalculia.* We see much less of this, perhaps because it is rarer. More likely it is because arithmetic is less important than reading. A child can fail arithmetic and be promoted, if his other grades are good. A person can go through life severely handicapped in his ability to calculate and simply plan his life around it. He can be a philosopher, clergyman, physician, and a thousand other occupations. But if a child has a neurological dysfunction that prohibits him from reading well, then he is in serious trouble. He can't even be a mathematician, because he cannot read the problems he could otherwise calculate.

Since reading and writing, with the exception just noted, are the only basic neurological processes taught in school, we feel information about brain function is essential to the teaching of them. We submit that educators, in their earnest endeavors to solve the reading problem, would find their attempts more rewarding if they would inject information about brain function into their consideration.

Educators would discover, for example, that the advocates of phonics and look-say are both right and both wrong, that if a child is normal—neurologically, intellectually, culturally and emotionally—he will learn to read regardless of the method used to teach him, but if he has dyslexia, neither method will be wholly satisfactory.

When information about brain function is added to the educational mix, reading specialists will begin to understand what they do not presently know, that is, how the normal child actually goes about the neurological process of reading. More importantly, they will discover how this process breaks down because of perceptual impairments to create problem readers. And they will begin to see some possible ways to improve or bypass these debilitating impairments.

With the addition of information about brain function, teachers and school administrators will start to see the proper way to amalgamate both phonics and look-say into the reading program, how and when to teach silent reading for meaning, the importance of spelling and other factors. Most vitally, educators can stop unproductive controversies about phonics versus look-say and the value of educational research and the various causes of reading disorders. With knowledge of brain function, all of these controversies are beside the point. To be sure, controversies will still exist after educators are armed with the needed information. They will be able to argue whether basal readers, language experience or individualized learning is the best method of instruction, whether one system of instructional materials is better, and many other matters. But at least these controversies will be more productive than the present ones.

We are not suggesting for a moment that neurological information is a magic cure-all for the ills of education. We are not saying that all the problem readers will disappear. On the contrary, the problems of dyslexia we present are most difficult to solve and will be with us for a very long time. All we are saying is that when a neurologist looks at reading, the ignorance of educators about brain function is most apparent and that without that information they cannot remove children from the wayside of education.

PART TWO

A NEUROLOGIST LOOKS AT READING

3.
A New Definition of Reading

WHEN A NEUROLOGIST looks at reading as it is taught in the United States, he finds confusion about what reading is. Some teachers are laboring under a definition of reading that makes the task more difficult than it needs to be—and it isn't easy at best.

WHAT IS READING?

Over and over, in book after book, authority upon authority maintains that reading is gaining the meaning of the words written on a page. A typical example is from *Reading in Child Development* by Professor William H. Burton of Harvard. He says the process of reading is commonly defined as (his italics) *"getting meaning from the printed page."* A more accurate definition is *"bringing meaning to the printed page."*[1]

Also typical is the writing of Paul McKee, who says there are three major acts in reading: (1) identifying and recognizing printed words quickly and accurately; (2) arriving at an adequate understanding of meaning intended by the writer; and (3) making use of the meaning arrived at.[2]

Dr. Kathleen B. Hester, Professor of Education at Eastern Michigan University, asks, "What then is reading? Some people believe that it is reading words of a page and not getting the thought of an author." She maintains that if teachers accept this definition and teach accordingly, future generations will not have learned to evaluate. They will be ready victims for propaganda.

Professor Hester says, "Reading in its real sense involves both . . . recognition of words and getting the thought of an author. In addition, it involves critical and creative thinking. A student must relate what he reads to his own experiences. He must interpret and evaluate the material, exercise reason and imagination and fuse new ideas with previous learnings to gain power to think independently. Not until he can carry on these complex thought processes as he reads can he classify himself as a good reader."[3]

We suggest that Professor Hester has given a most appealing definition, not of reading, but of *education.*

The idea that one has not read until he understands the meaning of the words printed on the page is the fundamental concept, the cornerstone, of reading instruction in this country. The principal criticism leveled at phonics by the advocates of the look-say method is that phonics teaches "word calling" and not reading. The child who is expert in phonics learns to pronounce a great many words the meaning of which he does not know. He can word-call, but cannot read, the look-sayers insist. He is illiterate.

We will not dispute that the ultimate aim of reading is to enable the readers to obtain an idea from an author with all his nuances of meaning. But the ultimate aim of speech and hearing is also to communicate. Reading is but one means of communication, a tool by which human beings exchange ideas and information.

From a neurological standpoint, *reading is translating graphic symbols into SOUND according to a recognized system.*

THREE LEVELS OF READING

When a child goes to school to learn to read, he has an auditory vocabulary variously estimated at between 2,500 and 20,000 words, depending on his intelligence, his maturity and the environment to which he has been exposed.

In school the teacher writes on the blackboard, or points to a page, on which is written some funny scribbles. The teacher tells the child the scribbles say, "Run." He looks at the scribbles carefully and accepts the teacher's word for it that those three scribbles are *run*. He knows what *run* means. He has heard the word thousands of times. He has run for miles. He is an expert on running. He looks at the word again. Those scribbles mean *run* and for the rest of his life they will mean *run*.

Neurologically, this child had, before he ever appeared at school, a network established, and well established, so that the sound of the word *run*, received by his ear and converted to nerve impulses, was sent to an area or areas of the brain whose function is language comprehension. He evaluated the context in which *run* was used and either ran or did not run or ran fast or slowly or to a certain point in accordance with the full instructions.

Now, confronted with the word *run*, it is a simple process—if he has no impairment in his perception—for him to hook a visual link to his existing sound network. What he actually does is sound out the word *run*, which has meaning for him. In this beginning, first level of reading, he actually utters aloud every word he sees and listens to himself saying it. He is using the sound-to-comprehension network which he began to establish in his infancy and which is well formulated by the time he enters the first grade. His task in the first grade is to start to establish a sight-to-sound-to-comprehension system.

With practice, this new network becomes more efficient, and he reaches the second level of reading, wherein the sight of a word automatically tells him its sound and thus its meaning. He no longer has to hear the word uttered. He hears mentally, although he may actually say it silently to himself so that measurable vibrations are set up in his vocal cords. He is like a person who is rehearsing a speech, actually hears himself making his remarks although no sound escapes his lips. Neurologically, the second-level reading is still making use of his infantile sound-to-comprehension network, but he has added a sight link. He has become so adept at going from sight to sound to comprehension that the whole process is automatic and quite rapid.

The overwhelming majority of readers do this for the rest of their lives. The ranks of readers who mentally sound out every word they will ever read includes presidents, generals, eminent scholars and teachers of remedial reading. It is a perfectly acceptable and most advantageous method of reading. It is a somewhat slower method, but it permits the person to savor the words he reads, to enjoy style and rhythm of fine writing.

There is a third level of reading reached by a small percentage of people, wherein the sound of the word is eliminated entirely and the person goes directly from the graphic symbol to the meaning. He reads rapidly, gaining the thought and information represented by the words on the page. It is an asset because of its speed, but can be a curse in that the stylistic virtues of the writing are often lost on him. He is often a heavy-handed writer.

Some people can learn to read at the third level by practice, although many are never able to become accomplished at it no matter how hard they try. There are some, too, who can do both second- and third-level reading and thus enjoy the pleasures of both worlds.*

The teacher of reading in the primary grades should not be concerned with training the third-level reader. He must teach him the first level, translating marks on paper into sound, and get him into the second level, wherein the process becomes more rapid and automatic. If he later reaches the third level, fine, but it is not something to be taught—nor can it be learned in the first three grades.

There is a simile which may further clarify the difference between second- and third-level reading. The second-level reader is like the high-school student or adult who studies French. In the beginning, this person mentally translates the French into English which he understands. With practice, this French student becomes like the third-level reader and actually understands the French without making the translation into English. Thus, the second-level reader translates graphic symbols into sound which he understands and, with practice, may learn to gain meaning from the printed words without translating them into sound.

The neurologists' message about the importance of sound in the reading process is beginning to get through to educators. Dr.

---

* It must be suspected that John F. Kennedy was such an individual. By all reports he was a most rapid reader, able to devour great quantities of written material in such a short time that it amazed his associates. At the same time, he was an obvious stylist, able to put thoughts on paper in an artistic manner.

Helen B. Carey of the Philadelphia Public Schools wrote in "The Bright Underachiever in Reading. Causes of Underachievement":

> Recently, a new group has made itself very much heard. It comprises the advocates of what is referred to as the linguistic approach to the teaching of reading. On this subject the linguists have much to say to which we should be well-advised to listen. If everything they claim is correct, then much that has so far been done in our schools is incorrect, and many of us have been working hard to produce underachievers.
>
> The linguists claim first of all that reading is a double perceptual process. Language is speech and the written or printed symbol is a symbol for a speech sound, not for a concept. When we read, we perceive first the written word as a symbol for sound, and then perceive the sound as a symbol for the concept. So-called vocalization or sub-vocalization is not an unusual phenomenon characterizing the reading of the very young child, and later the inefficient slow reader—it is well-nigh universal. Experiments with electronic devices attached to the throat have indicated that sub-vocalization takes place with practically every reader, no matter how skillful and rapid he may be.[4]

READING AND COMPREHENSION

It is important for the teacher to realize that translating marks on paper into sounds is reading and is one function of the brain. Comprehending the meaning of those sounds is a different function of the brain.

If the teacher were to pick up a textbook on neurosurgery and read every word in it, chances are he would find it rather difficult. It would be filled with physiology and anatomy and medical terms unfamiliar to him. When he was finished, he would say, "I read every word of this textbook on neurosurgery, but I didn't understand it." He differentiates between reading and comprehension, yet turns around and decries the fact that one of his pupils, while able to orally read "Run, Spot, Run," doesn't comprehend that Spot is a dog and that the meaning of the words is for the dog to get a move on. This pupil has a serious problem in comprehension, but he reads well.*

* The State of Connecticut, among others, requires a registering voter to prove he can read. The registrar hands the registrant a paper on which are

Comprehension of both the spoken and written word is a matter of intelligence, age and maturity, and experience. A person's comprehension increases by seeing and hearing and doing and feeling and continues through his entire life, as he gains information and concepts and relates them to his previous experience and "thinks" about life and problems and situations. Comprehension involves interacting with other people and becoming involved in situations.

A major method of increasing comprehension, of course, is by reading. A child translates a mark on paper into a sound that has meaning for him. As his efficiency improves, he learns the marks that symbolize all the words in his oral vocabulary, then goes on to obtain a reading vocabulary that far exceeds his oral vocabulary. He learns information and concepts which enable him to comprehend still more material *ad infinitum.*

A most important task of the teacher, perhaps *the* most important, is to improve the child's comprehension. He teaches him geography and history, health and science, arithmetic and government. He takes him on trips to the zoo and the museum, shows him movies of far-off places, invites lecturers to speak to him, and much, much more, all of it designed to increase his comprehension. He tries to instill in him a love of comprehension, for this is the lifelong process of education.

The teacher also teaches him to *read,* to translate a mark on paper into sound by a recognized system, for this is a vital tool by which his comprehension is increased.

The difference between reading and comprehension can be illustrated by an analogy from a military situation. A message comes in by radio in Morse code. The radioman listens to the sound of the dots and dashes and translates them into letters which he writes on a piece of paper. But when he finishes taking the entire message, he cannot understand the message because it had been sent in cryptographic code. The message was just a jumble of letters and numbers that had no meaning to him.

The radioman takes the message to the intelligence officer, who

---

typed about ten words, taken out of context, from the middle of the state constitution. Reciting the words is legal proof of the ability to read. The actual sentence, according to a recent registrant, is virtually devoid of meaning.

gets out his code book and translates the message into understandable English and takes appropriate action.

From a neurological standpoint, the radioman "read" and the intelligence officer "comprehended" meaning. The teacher is endeavoring to train both radiomen and intelligence officers. The task is more difficult because he cannot teach the child to be an intelligence officer until he teaches him to be a radioman *first*. By understanding the separate functions of the brain, even though it is not usually practical to teach the functions separately, we believe the teacher can better understand the difficulties of the beginning reader.

Carrying the military analogy further, we can grasp some other functions of the brain. The "input radioman" reads and passes the message to the "intelligence officer," who would like to send a message in reply; the intelligence officer then uses a second "output radioman," who transmits messages by writing. Writing uses language comprehension (the same intelligence officer).

Understanding the separate functions of the brain allows a teacher to realize why a student can be a good reader and a poor speller or why word recognition may be poor and comprehension good or why oral and silent reading ability may differ in the same individual. Simple observation of these phenomena should enable the teacher to grasp the root of the problem and perhaps plan a more precise remedial reading program.

If we apply our military analogy to auditory as distinct from visual language, we can envision the same basic arrangement. There is a radioman for receiving (sensory) speech, the same old intelligence officer for language comprehension and another radioman for sending (motor) speech. And we have the same possibilities for difficulties—a child who understands what is said to him, but cannot speak so others can comprehend him; or a child who cannot understand what is said to him but has peerless diction when uttering jargon.

We have endeavored to illustrate these various links between visual and auditory perception, language comprehension and motor ability with diagrams.

Preparing such diagrams is difficult because these functions are complex. So many brain functions are involved that fully accurate diagrams would resemble the proverbial Chinese puzzles. Regardless of this, we believe there may be value in attempting to illustrate some of the processes we have discussed in this chapter.

To understand these diagrams it is necessary to discard some popular notions. First, the ears and the eyes are merely implements for gathering sound waves and registering visual impressions. We hear and see with the brain. Second, not all functions of the brain are localized. Evidence indicates that the "centers" of hearing are in one particular area and vision is centered in another. Certain other functions have been localized. But researchers have had little success in efforts to localize such functions as language comprehension, reading, writing, calculation or various forms of perception. We know these functions exist, but whether they are performed in one area of the brain or in several has not been accurately determined. In these drawings we have tried to differentiate by boxing the localized functions and encircling the nonlocalized.

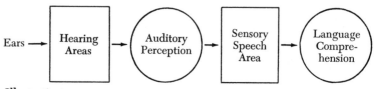

Illustration 2

Illustration 2 shows an important pre-reading function the normal child possesses when he enters the first grade. The ear picks up the sound waves uttered by the teacher. Nerve impulses are created which are transferred through a complex network to the "hearing areas." Next, auditory perception is used so the specific sounds uttered by the teacher are distinguished from all other possible sounds. Going next to the area for sensory-speech function, the sounds perceived are recognized as those of specific words uttered by the teacher. These sounds are then checked for meaning by language comprehension, and the child, having heard and recognized the teacher's words, comes to comprehend their meaning. Everyone uses this process everytime he hears a spoken word. It is such a rapid process that we fail to realize these step-by-step functions have taken place. For the very young child, the process is much more deliberate, as it is with an adult learning a foreign language.

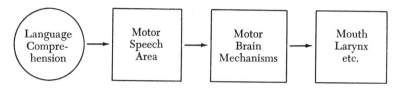

Illustration 3

Illustration 3 shows another important pre-reading function of the normal child. He is able to speak, a process that goes from language comprehension to motor speech, to the appropriate motor areas and then to the mouth, tongue, larynx and other apparatus for speaking.

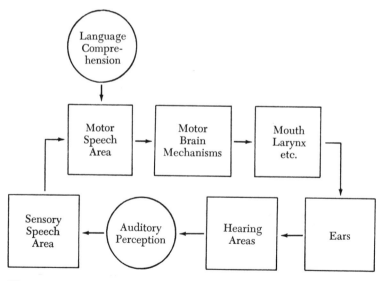

Illustration 4

By combining the first two diagrams (see Illustration 4) we can see how one listens to his own speech and thereby corrects his own errors or learns to make new sounds correctly.

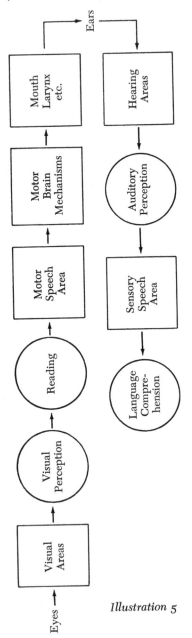

Illustration 5

Illustration 5 is a representation of the first level of reading. The image on the page is picked up by the eyes, transferred to the visual areas in the brain. Then, in visual perception the individual letters are distinguished from all other marks. Next, the reading function occurs, in which the child recognizes that which he has perceived to be a word and compares it to other known word images to identify it. At this point he says the word aloud, going through the functions of motor-speech. He then hears himself say the word and makes use of his long-established ability to hear, recognize and comprehend the spoken word. This is a tortuous route to language comprehension, but this is what the beginning reader does in order to make use of his existing neurological abilities.

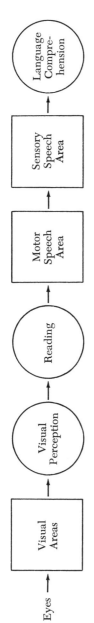

Illustration 6 is the second level of reading used by most individuals all of the time and all individuals some of the time. In this diagram we are trying to convey the fact that the person eliminates the mechanics of motor-speech. He no longer says the word aloud and hears himself say it, although vibrations may be set up in his larynx and some portions of the mechanics of speech take place. But certainly the brain function of motor-speech occurs. He goes through the mental process of saying the word without actually uttering it, and similarly he uses the hearing or sensory-speech function without using his ears and temporal cortex in order to reach language comprehension. This is still an involved process, but considerably shortened from the first stage of reading.

Illustration 6

The third level of reading reached by a small minority of rapid readers is shown in Illustration 7. Here the person goes directly from visual perception to language comprehension, omitting any reference to the sound of the word. A new pathway to language comprehension has been established which permits rapid reading for meaning

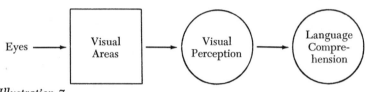

Illustration 7

By combining the previous diagrams (see Illustration 8), one can illustrate the development that occurs as a child progresses through the levels of reading.

Reading is a tool to language comprehension as Illustration 9 indicates. Language comprehension occurs through the ears by listening, through the sense of touch, as well as through vision. The normal child will certainly benefit if all three routes are used, if he hears words said and writes them. If a child is dyslexic and has an impairment of one form of perception, greater use must be made of the other forms of perception in order to reach language comprehension. In the school setting, visual imperception occurs most often and causes the greatest difficulty, thus indicating the great value of phonic training in remedial programs. It should be pointed out that this illustration does not show that the auditory portion of reading comes first in all three pathways. It may be possible to learn reading without sound, but this is very rare. For virtually everyone, language must be learned auditorily before any language can be read.

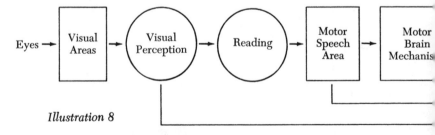

Illustration 8

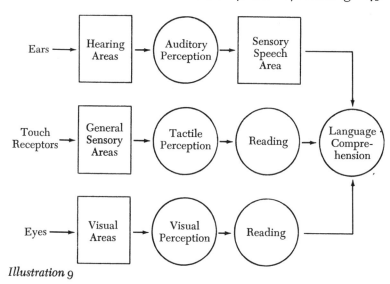

Illustration 9

When first learning to read, the child is concentrating so hard on the *reading* process that he bypasses language comprehension and goes directly on to the speech mechanism. In Illustration 10, the child reads aloud with no comprehension of what is read. This is normal at first. If this state continues into the second and third grades, the child should be studied to find why he continues to bypass comprehension.

Illustration 11 represents a pathway we all have used—sensory-speech to writing without comprehension. This is the mechanism that is in action when we take notes at a lecture but have little or no understanding of the subject until we read the material over again. This is often the pathway used in spelling tests in elementary-school pupils.

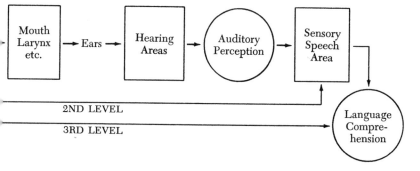

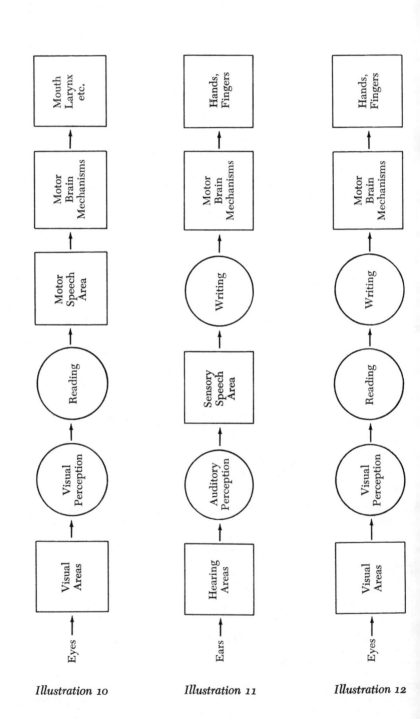

Illustration 10   *Illustration 11*   *Illustration 12*

Illustration 12 shows a mechanism that is obviously present—and yet demonstrates the separation of reading from comprehension. This is the mechanism of copying a known or an unknown language. This is also the mechanism of visual control of our writing—working unconsciously whenever we write. If you don't think this is necessary, close your eyes the next time you write a letter.

When one understands that reading is translating a mark on paper into sound, he begins to realize some of the problems of the dyslexic child. If the dyslexic child has poor visual perception, he has difficulty recognizing the mark on paper, and if he has auditory imperception, he does not correctly discriminate the sound represented. His problem can range from virtually total inability to simple slowness which makes it difficult for him to keep pace with his classmates.

When one understands that reading and comprehension are different functions of the brain, he understands that a dyslexic child can be a poor reader yet have excellent comprehension. He learns orally and in all ways except by reading. There is no reason that he should be tossed to the wayside because he is a poor reader. He can learn information and become quite productive in life.

In reality, the dyslexic child has more problems than translating a mark on paper into sound, for reading is the most complex neurological task a person undertakes in his lifetime. That human beings are able to read at all is a miracle. Yet, most of us are able to do it so effortlessly that we fail to realize how difficult it is. As we point out some of these difficulties in the next chapter, we might keep in mind that the dyslexic child knows how difficult reading is. He is an expert on that subject.

4.

Reading Is a Complex Task

WHEN A CHILD IS SIX, he goes to school and learns to read—if he is not dyslexic. In reality, several complicated neurological and psychological processes have gone on before which enable the normal child to read. A brief look at these processes will help us understand why a normal child is able to master the difficult art of reading and some of the reasons that the dyslexic child fails.

BRAIN MATURATION

Chronologically, the first and most vital process which must occur if the child is to learn to read, or anything else, is brain maturation. The progress the individual child makes in this process determines to a large degree his success in learning to roll over, sit up, walk, talk, read and master Einstein's Theory of Relativity. In instructing the first-grader to read, it is essential that his teacher realize he is working with a developing, not an adult brain.

Parents and teachers are aware that a child's physical and intellectual abilities develop in a sequential manner. He sits at six months, begins to talk at 12 months, reads at six years and so on. There is a pronounced tendency to blame all failure in school performance on "immaturity."

While nearly everyone has observed a child's developing maturity, relatively few people have understood why this is so. The reason a child's ability, both intellectual and motor, develops so slowly is that he must await the maturation of the cells in his brain. Every normal human being is born with a full complement of brain cells. He has, at his birth, every cell he will ever own. If any of these cells is destroyed by an injury or illness, he will never replace it. The body has no mechanism to grow new brain cells.

When a baby is born, the vast majority of his brain cells are unusable. If one looks at the nerve cells in a newborn's brain, he will observe that the cells are of different shape and size than those of an adult.

The process of brain maturation can be followed by watching cell change. The cells grow in size, assume a different shape and chemical composition. The framework on which the cells are hung also grows, and the size of the head containing the brain enlarges. This process goes on for roughly 18 years, after which an individual will have a fully mature brain, in the neurophysiological sense. His learning will continue for the rest of his life, as he uses and expands the uses of the functions with which Nature provided him.

The neurological maturation of the brain goes on generally in a logical sequence and at a regular rate. At first it is quite rapid. A three-year-old has about 90 percent of his ultimate brain size. After that the rate of cell growth slows as maturity becomes more conceptual and less physical.

Neurological maturation is important in the educational process, because children's brains do not mature at the same rate. We know that some children sit up at six months, but others not until a later age. Some babies walk at nine months and others don't develop the capacity until 15 or 16 months.

In infancy, these discrepancies in developmental schedules don't matter much. The child sits, walks, talks, and goes into training pants eventually. But when he becomes six, he goes to school—by law. He must learn to read, whether he is neurologically mature or not. If he doesn't, he fails the first grade, falls behind in the educational derby right at the start and may never catch up. He may not go to college and perhaps will miss the brass ring of life.

Every teacher has observed this child. He seems intelligent and he tries to learn, but he just doesn't catch on to what reading is all about. Then, all of a sudden in the second semester of the first grade or in the second or third year of school, he grasps it. The whole process of reading becomes magically simple.

It is important that two points be made here. First, the finer the neurological process, the greater the disparity in its development among children. The time span in which normal children learn to sit up is relatively shorter than the time span in which normal children learn to walk. The span widens as children learn to talk and it grows quite wide with the acquisition of the more difficult English sounds. One normal child may learn to say the *r* sound, for example, a year or two later than another normal child. The developmental discrepancy between normal children is at its widest in reading and writing. One normal child may be able to read at five years of age and another normal child at seven. It is important in the educational process that teachers expect a far greater variance in neurological maturation for reading and writing than for running or walking or climbing stairs.

The second major point we wish to make is that, while there is a relationship between reading and other forms of neurological maturation, it is not a causal relationship. A child who has been consistently tardy in sitting, walking, talking, running, climbing stairs, and abandoning diapers may be expected to be somewhat slower in his neurological maturation for reading, but the fact that he was tardy about his infant and preschool development is not a *reason* that he is a delayed reader. A parent, teacher or physician might surmise upon becoming aware of a child's history of slow neurological development that he is slow in reading maturation, but it is a gross mistake to assume that the way to speed up his maturation for reading is to drill him in preschool activities. A theory exists that there is a relationship between motor ability and the ability to discriminate shapes and patterns by reading. According to this theory, if a child who is a poor reader performs various physical exercises his reading will improve. From a neurological standpoint, the way the brain is made precludes any possible relationship between motor and visual abilities. This has been difficult to prove, however, in a clinical or educational setting. If the motor training goes on long enough, natural brain maturation may lead to improvement in reading. It has been difficult to show, however, that it is a natural process and not the motor exercises that produces the improvement.

However, we now have a careful study on motor training by Coralie Dietrich, a psychologist at the University of Wisconsin at Stevens Point. Ms. Dietrich took forty-four children between the ages of seven and eleven, all of whom were of normal to high IQ yet were in the lower half of their age groups in reading. At random the children were placed in three groups. One group received daily motor training. The second received daily individualized remedial reading instruction. The third was a control group performing general activities. At the end of six months, the various groups were evaluated in terms of improved reading performance. Ms. Dietrich reported her findings in these words:

> The perceptual motor training had no significant effect on reading achievement; in fact this group performed more poorly in reading than either of the other two groups. . . . Perceptual motor training was also not effective in bringing about significant changes in perceptual motor development itself. . . . The perceptual motor training group's significantly poorer performance on the school behavior variables does not support the notion that the playful non-academic atmosphere and simple attentional elements involved in these programs help children with their school adjustment and learning problems. . . . Finally, the total analyses suggest that in terms of the main problem addressed in this investigation, the perceptual motor training techniques examined here are in fact one of the "panaceas" referred to by Kass (1969), and are particularly fruitless and unfortunate approaches for the remediation of reading problems. This study suggests that for both the child's development in problem reading areas and behavior adjustment, the more arduous road of long term individualized remedial reading instruction is the answer.[1]

Brain maturation is without doubt a major factor in dyslexia. We cannot indiscriminately open heads and examine the brain cells of these youngsters, but the empirical evidence of the number of children whose dyslexia is transient in nature is quite striking. Many children who have perceptual difficulties at age six show considerable improvement by age ten or 12. Some of this improvement may be due to training and experience, but most of it results from brain maturation. This characteristic of dyslexia should be considered in any program of educational therapy.

READING READINESS

Coincidental with the neurological process of maturation is the psychological process of readiness. Teachers are most familiar with the concept of readiness, but an understandable confusion often exists between maturation and readiness.

A person may be neurologically mature, but he is not ready to learn calculus because he has not mastered arithmetic and algebra. A first-grader may have the neurological capacity to read, but not be ready to read because of insufficient preschool experiences or insufficient discipline in sitting still, listening and studying.

The distinction between maturation and readiness has been aptly made by psychologist David P. Ausubel:

> There is little disagreement about the fact that readiness always crucially influences the efficiency of the learning process and often determines whether a given intellectual skill or type of school material is learnable at all at a particular stage of development. Most educators also implicitly accept the proposition that an age of readiness exists for every kind of learning. Postponement of learning experience beyond this age of readiness wastes valuable and often unsuspected learning opportunities, thereby unnecessarily reducing the amount and complexity of subject-matter content that can be mastered in a designated period of schooling. On the other hand, when a pupil is prematurely exposed to a learning task before he is ready for it, he not only fails to learn the task in question but also learns from the experience of failure, to fear, dislike and avoid it. . . .
>
> Difficulty first arises when it [readiness] is confused with the concept of maturation, and when the latter concept in turn is equated with the process of "internal ripening." The concept of readiness simply refers to the adequacy of existing capacity in relation to the demands of a given learning task. No specification is made to *how* this capacity is achieved—whether through prior practice of a specific nature (learning), through incidental experience, through genetically regulated structural and functional changes occurring independently of environmental influences, or through various combinations of these factors. Maturation, on the other hand, has a different and much more restricted meaning. It encompasses those increments in capacity that take place in the demonstrable absence of specific practice experience, i.e., that are attributable to genetic influence and/or incidental experience. Maturation, therefore, is not the same as readiness but is merely one of the two principal factors (the other being learning) that contribute to or determine the organism's readiness to cope with

new experience. Whether or not readiness exists, in other words, does not necessarily depend on maturation alone but in many instances is solely a function of prior learning experience and most typically depends on varying proportions of maturation and learning.[2]

Then Dr. Ausubel makes this important point:

> To equate the principles of readiness and maturation not only muddies the conceptual waters, but also makes it difficult for the school to appreciate that insufficient readiness may reflect inadequate prior learning on the part of pupils because of inappropriate or inefficient instructional methods. Lack of maturation can thus become a conveniently available scapegoat whenever children manifest insufficient readiness to learn; and the school, which is thereby automatically absolved of all responsibility in the matter, consequently fails to subject its instructional practices to the degree of self-critical scrutiny necessary for continued educational progress. In short, while it is important to appreciate that the current readiness of pupils determines the school's current choice of instructional methods and materials, it is equally important to bear in mind that this readiness itself is partly determined by the appropriateness and efficiency of the previous instructional practices to which they have been subjected.

To paraphrase Dr. Ausubel, you can't learn calculus without algebra. He goes on to discuss the influence of environment on "internal ripening," saying that "unique factors of individual experience and cultural environment make important contributions to the direction, patterning, and sequential order of all developmental changes." It is a mistake, he maintains, to assume that environmental factors do not influence maturation.

> It is hardly surprising, therefore, in view of the tremendous influence on professional and lay opinion wielded by Gesell and his colleagues, that many people conceive of readiness in absolute and immutable terms, and thus fail to appreciate that except for such traits as walking and grasping, the mean age of readiness can never be specified apart from relevant environmental conditions. Although the model child in contemporary America may first be ready to read at the age of six and one-half, the age of reading readiness is always influenced by cultural, subcultural, and individual differences in background experience, and in any case varies with the method of instruction employed and the child's

IQ. Middle-class children, for example, are ready to read at an earlier age than lower-class children because of the greater availability of books in the home, and because they are "read to" and "taken places" more frequently.

We have quoted Dr. Ausubel at length in hopes it will negate any tendency on the part of parents and teachers to assume that neurological immaturity is the *only* cause of a child's failure to read. It *may* be a factor, along with environmental influences, poor previous learning experiences and other matters affecting reading readiness.

SPEECH

The child entering the first grade to learn to read must have sufficient brain maturation and he must be psychologically ready to read. He must also have speech, for since reading is translating marks on paper into sound, he must be an expert in oral and auditory language.

Writing—that is, material which is read—is printed speech, a permanent method of recording speech. This statement should not be construed to mean that all utterances should be written down or that all writing is intended to be read aloud. The nuances of meaning which the human voice can give to speech, nuances impossible to duplicate in printed speech, have through the years led to development of stylistic techniques in writing words to be spoken which differ from those used in writing words to be read silently. But the fact remains that, because we sound out every word we read (or write), we are producing, in writing, a permanent record of speech. Writing follows speech, whether or not the writing is ever uttered aloud, and therefore speech is the key to writing.

Human speech is such a complex, precise function that one could not believe that a child 24 months of age could accomplish it, if he did not hear it happening regularly. Speaking in sentences is at least as difficult for a child of that age as playing a Beethoven violin concerto. This toddler, who may still be having difficulty walking and certainly cannot walk down stairs efficiently, learns to coordinate movements of his tongue, soft palate, respiratory processes, jaws, and facial muscles so expertly and smoothly that he can produce intelligible speech. More than producing the sounds of his native language, he learns at an early age to organize the sounds into words, sentences and paragraphs. He can use those organized sounds to relate information and to report concepts. By the time he is two years old, the child will have passed through, according to psychologist Dorothea Mc-Carthy,[3] 126 language steps from grunts to the use of certain prepositions. By the time he is an undergraduate in college, he will have an oral vocabulary estimated at between 100,000 and 200,000 words![4]

For the child, learning to speak is a leisurely process taking a half dozen years or more for full development. He is given ample opportunity to learn by trial and error, and he receives a minimum of didactic instruction. He begins in his crib by making sounds best described as grunts, coos and gurgles. These sounds are probably related to his functional ability. As maturation occurs in his nervous system, his ability to make sounds improves, and the sounds he makes are evidence of his brain maturation.

We can synopsize the lengthy process of speech development by saying the child begins by making random sounds consisting of a vowel and later a consonant. In time he repeats these first sounds and says "Dada." This sound gains him a pleasant reaction from other members of his family, particularly the adult male member. The baby discovers that when he says "Dada" he is fussed over, talked to, smiled at and picked up. He deduces that this sound must be important and have meaning. He discovers in time that other sounds he babbles fail to achieve this reaction, but that some, such as "Papa," "Mama" and "Bye bye" do have meaning. Eventually he discards the meaningless sounds to the point that he forgets how to make them. Thus, the Chinese baby discards the *l* sound, which does not exist in his language. Parents, siblings and others are teaching the child by an inductive method those sounds which are important. At the same time he is learning concepts, that "Dada" refers to one particular male and not to all men he meets, that "Bye bye" gets him taken out in his carriage and is not a term that brings him a bottle.

This process of making sounds, reinforcement and concept goes on for years. He learns to make nonrepetitive sounds such as "Baby," then increasingly complex words, phrases, sentences and paragraphs. Under constant reinforcement and instruction from his family, he learns to comprehend meaning and express his own thoughts. He learns grammar, syntax, the sequential order of language, concepts and much more. That he accomplishes speech is in part a tribute to his motivation. He wants to learn to speak and works quite hard at it. His parents want him to speak, for it is (to them) a mark of his intelligence, so they offer him a great deal of help and encouragement. They are most patient with him. It is a pleasant time for both parents and child.

With few exceptions, hearing is essential to speech. The exceptions are deaf children who are now taught to speak, some of them quite well, in most school systems. But teaching deaf children to speak is a most difficult, time-consuming task, involving special mockups that show the child the position of the tongue, palate and lips and enable him to judge the amount of air to be expelled and the vibrations associated with correct speech. Furthermore the deaf child must be shown everything. He must see an apple, for it cannot be described to him.

The amazing case, of course, is Helen Keller, who could neither see nor hear, yet learned to speak and to read Braille entirely through the sense of touch. She felt the apple and the raised dots on paper that meant apple and the vibrations in the throat and the movement of the lips when the word *apple* was uttered. She had heard language and spoken a few words before her illness, yet that she was able to learn to speak and read is almost beyond belief.

READING IS HARDER THAN SPEAKING

This brief description of the manner in which a child learns to speak has been provided because, in learning to read, the child recapitulates much of the process. He learns letters instead of vowel and consonant sounds, discovering that graphic letters on a page represent the sounds which he utters. He learns to put together consonants and vowels to make words, such as *run*. He learns to put -*ner* or -*ning* on the end to read *runner* or *running*, in the manner in which linguists such as Dr. Fries have pointed out. He learns more complex words, and phrases, sentences and paragraphs, much as he does in speaking. He undergoes constant instruction by the teacher and so learns which pronunciation is correct and has meaning. He discovers concepts to be derived from those graphic symbols on the page.

But reading is vastly more difficult than speech. First of all, the rules under which he learns to read are drastically changed. For four and a half years, since he learned to walk and talk, he has been urged to run and play, to go outdoors, to be active. If he looks at a book for other than a few minutes a day, his parents suspect there is something wrong with him and urge him to go out and exercise. Then suddenly, in the sixth year of his life, his mother tears August off the calendar and he is sent to school, where emphasis is not on running and playing, but on sitting still, listening, doing what he is told and something known as "study-ing," a concept with which he is not too familiar. The first-grader discovers rather painfully that his freedom is sharply curtailed. His life, at least one third of the day for nine months a year, is quite regimented. This takes some getting used to.

But the biggest rule change is in the manner in which he is taught to read and write as against the way he learned verbal language. Gone is the leisurely pace, the feeling of abundant time, the opportunity for trial and error, the luxury of self-discovery. The teacher does not invite him to attempt to write the word *run* and let him try until he discovers how to do it. The first time he tried he might produce a square, a triangle and circle and happily go to the teacher declaring it to be *run*. She says that in English squares and triangles, two of the most common, easily understood forms to the first-grader, do not exist. The circle is all right, but it isn't found in *run*. Chances are that, if the teacher waited long enough, this hypothetical first-grader would acciden-tally discover how to write *run* and the rest of the English language and, if the teacher were patient, it would be as much fun for both teacher and student as learning speech is for parents and offspring.

But in school there isn't time for such luxurious trial and error. The first-grader must learn rules and prescribed limits, ways that are correct, methods that are approved. If he commits errors, he receives a bad grade, extra work or is moved back into the third reading group. If he fails, he repeats the grade and suffers the parental disapproval and the ridicule of his peers. In short, there is a punitive aspect to learning to read and write that never existed when the child learned to speak. The pressure for performance is on and will last for the rest of his life.

Our point here is not to criticize the rules, procedures or even the pressure. This is part of life and a child must learn it. The rules are often necessary if the child is to profit from his quite expensive education. All we are suggesting is that there is some value in understanding that reading is a recapitulation of speech performed under far more difficult circumstances.

Another, more important reason that reading is harder to learn than speech is that reading is a double code, while speech is a single code. In speech a child translates a sound into meaning. In reading, the child translates a mark on paper first into sound and second into meaning. The task he is learning is comparable to learning Morse code. A radio operator receives dots and dashes, translates them into letters, which he makes into words that are sounds, and which then become meaning, really a triple code. After he becomes adept, the telegrapher ceases to hear individual letters for the most part and listens in syllables and whole words. The cryptographer uses much the same process.

We are teaching a child a most difficult process in reading. We seldom realize how difficult it is. Reading is a visual form of speech, but the typesetter is not so efficient as the human voice. In written language, we have no way to reflect intonation of speech. We try, with punctuation, italics and capitalization, but these are at best only the poorest substitutes for the human voice. When we speak in anger, we can make our anger felt, not so much in our choice of words, but in the tone with which we deliver them. The same words, when written, can convey anger only with the greatest difficulty. The writer must, with considerable talent, establish an entire scene with characters and elaborate past developments so that the reader knows that anger is the proper emotion in the present circumstance. We have no way, in reading, as we have in speech, to convey the intent of the author. There is no symbol in English for disgust or hate or kindliness or insincerity or any other human emotion or attitude. Emotion and intent must be inferred from the graphic symbols on the page and it isn't at all easy. The same words can be read with many different meanings. Consider the sentence: "You brought me a glass of water." Is the speaker making a simple statement of fact? Or does he object that such a small amount was brought? Or is he surprised, dismayed or angered that the liquid is water rather than some other beverage? Or did he expect a steak dinner with all the trimmings? Or did he have in mind that someone else would bring the water? The list of possible interpretations of this simple sentence is far from exhausted. In reading we have to deduce this from the context. In speech there is no doubt what the speaker meant by the way he said it.

THE NATURE OF ENGLISH

Reading is truly difficult, a double code in which a graphic symbol is translated into sound. In making this definition of reading, we are referring, of course, to English. This definition also applies to a number of other languages, but not to all languages. The Japanese, for example, use a syllabary in which each Japanese character represents a syllable in the spoken language. American Indians used a pictographic language, in which simplified pictures were drawn to represent concepts, lightning for a storm, the sun for fair weather, etc.*

Then, there are ideographic languages, in which symbols or characters represent ideas or concepts. The symbols are not pictographic, but rather are quite arbitrary and must be learned. An example of an ideographic language is Chinese, a difficult language. Chinese has deteriorated somewhat from the pure ideographic with the adoption of some phonic characters. It is interesting that the Japanese adopted some of the Chinese characters, but used them to represent syllables rather than ideas.

Another interesting language is Egyptian hieroglyphics. It had no vowels. A sign could represent either a whole word or a part of a word. Hieroglyphics also used determinatives, that is, symbols appended to a sign that indicated the particular meaning intended.

English is an alphabetic language. Each character in the alphabet or combination of characters represents a sound in the English language, rather than a whole word, syllable or concept. An alphabetic language has several advantages. It is simple and most easily learned by children. There are relatively few charac-

* English writing has a few pictographic symbols in it, such as the dollar and cent signs, which are derived from a picture of a concept.

ters, and they stand consistently for the same sounds. Another advantage to an alphabetic language is that the alphabet can be used for more than one tongue. Thus, French, German, Italian, Portuguese, the Scandinavian tongues and several more use the same 26 characters that exist in English. Our alphabet has survived intact for 3,000 years, despite increased literacy, our rapidly growing vocabulary, and the invention of the printing press and the typewriter, which could have, but did not, corrupt the alphabet. Our alphabetic language is now receiving a new challenge from electronic data-processing equipment which "write" in dots and dashes and a host of other symbols that do not exist in our alphabet, but which the computer operator is trained to understand. How well the alphabet survives in the electronic era remains to be seen.

We submit that, despite its well-publicized imperfections, the English alphabet is a great advantage to us.* We should not abandon it—and we are in danger of doing it when the look-say method of reading is taught. The child learns not an alphabetic language—that is, alphabetic characters which stand for sounds —but graphic symbols which stand for a whole word or concept. He is urged to learn not the letters which represent the sounds of the word, but the configuration of the word as a whole.** That is the essence of an ideographic language, a technique much more akin to Chinese than English. The ideographic corruption of alphabetic English has been decried by famed linguist Leonard Bloomfield, who suggested such a method [look-say] loses all the advantages of an alphabetic language.[5]

Because speech is the key to reading, we can easily see how a child with auditory imperception will have immense difficulty. If

---

* We may have a great advantage in our alphabet, but we have great need for improvement in the use we make of it. Our language sorely needs systematizing. When we use the word *right,* for example, are we referring to a direction or indicating that something is correct? Such confusing idiosyncrasies were perhaps tolerable in more agricultural days, but in the scientific era such confusions are intolerable. It matters a great deal in a surgical operation, for example, if a term used to give a direction is misinterpreted to mean everything is "okay." There is something grossly ludicrous in a language in which *real* is a two-syllable word, while *ream* and *realm* are single-syllable words—with different vowel sounds. There are thousands of such confusions which must eventually be corrected—probably by government fiat. A commission of experts may have to be appointed someday to systematize English spelling.
** As will be shown later, the child does not do this.

he does not discriminate sounds correctly, he cannot speak correctly. So vital is auditory perception that children with moderate to severe auditory imperception never reach regular public school. Their speech difficulties are so gross that they are sent to special schools for aphasics. Some youngsters with mild imperception do reach regular public schools and we will discuss their problems in a subsequent chapter.

Oral and auditory language is a necessary framework for reading. The first addition to this framework involves sight or visual perception. The importance of this and the difficulties it poses for the dyslexic child are the subject of the next chapter.

5.

Recognizing the Marks on Paper

How DOES A CHILD learn to read? That millions accomplish the difficult task every year does not negate the fact that little is known about how the child does it. We strongly suspect that if an intelligent child who is neurologically, culturally and emotionally normal were left entirely to his own devices, but properly motivated to learn to read, he would discover how to do it himself. If given a few simple instructions, he would learn much more rapidly.

The vast majority of normal children will learn to read despite the methods of instruction used. It logically follows that if ideal teaching methods are used, the same child may learn more easily and at an earlier age. More importantly, the minority of children who are dyslexic may be helped over this necessary educational hurdle.

Some readers may be surprised that educators, psychologists and physicians do not know how a child learns to read. True, it is known that if a child is taught by a look-say method, phonic method, linguistics, augmented roman alphabet or some combination of these in a basal-reader, individualized or experience approach to teaching, he learns to read—or most of them do. But no one knows what goes on in a child's mind. How does he differentiate between letters? How does he translate the graphic symbol into sound? How does he group letters into combinations and words and sentences so the reading process becomes more rapid and automatic?

While our knowledge of how a child learns to read is far from complete, it is vastly extended as the result of a study performed at Cornell University, *A Basic Research Program on Reading*,[1] done in cooperation with the Office of Education of the U.S. Department of Health, Education, and Welfare. The two-and-a-half-inch-thick report which stemmed from the four-year study was released in 1963. Director of the project was Professor Harry Levin. Other faculty members, all psychologists, who performed and supervised the research, in which graduate students participated, were Eleanor J. Gibson, Alfred L. Baldwin, James J. Gibson, Charles F. Hockett, Henry N. Riccuiti and George J. Suci.

This is an excellent study. The research attempted was basic and the hypotheses tested were well thought out. The experiments to test the hypotheses were carefully designed and control groups were used to give an accurate measurement of the findings. Several studies were incomplete in their findings. We can only hope that the Cornell researchers or others will continue the work to a definitive conclusion. But the fact remains that the Cornell study was a highly scientific examination of how a child learns to read and, as such, a major contribution to the knowledge of reading and a tribute to Cornell University and its faculty. Unfortunately, copies of the full report are difficult to obtain. There is, however, an excellent evaluation of the findings by Eleanor Gibson in *Science*.[2]

We place great emphasis upon this study because it was obviously predicated upon knowledge of the neurological process of reading. The researchers had an awareness, for example, that reading is translating graphic symbols into sound, and the findings of the well-designed experiments provide the best indication so far of precisely how the child goes about this process. There are thousands of experimental studies which have been done to try to explain normal reading processes. The great majority of these are single isolated studies with little connection to the central problem, less applicability to teaching theory, and almost no neurological information. Many of these studies are poorly conceived and performed with inadequate control. It is neither necessary nor possible for this book to contain a critical review of this literature. The interested reader may find many excellent references in the Cornell study and may pursue the various subjects involved in the several indices available. While the results of the study are far from complete, we believe the Cornell study to be accurate, cohesive and most useful to the teacher and to the nonprofessional reader as well. We do not mean to imply that it is the only study, only that it is to our knowledge the best.

In her *Science* article, Dr. Gibson makes this statement: "Once a child begins his progression from spoken language to written language, there are, I think, three phases of learning to be considered. They present three different kinds of learning tasks, and they are roughly sequential, though there must be considerable overlapping. These three phases are: learning to differentiate graphic symbols; learning to decode letters to sounds ('map' the letters into sounds); and using progressively higher-order units of structure." The Cornell researchers set up experiments to explore each of these three stages.

Learning to differentiate each printed letter or number used in English is the first step in learning to read and it is not very easy. The same letter comes in various styles, such as capital and lower case, printed and cursive. There are a wide variety of typefaces, including *italic,* and a considerable range of sizes. When the letters are made by hand, as by a teacher, the variations both in printing and handwriting are endless and all of them vary in innumerable ways from printed letters.

PRESCHOOL TRAINING

The greatest difficulty for the beginning reader is that his preschool experiences may not have prepared him to discriminate between letters. For one thing, the child must discover the concept that an object (a letter) is not always the same regardless of its position. Nothing in his previous experience has prepared him for this. He knows, for example, that a golf club is a golf club no matter what its position or setting is. It's a golf club in his father's hand on the eighteenth fairway, in the golf bag in the closet, in the sporting goods store, whether new or damaged, backward or forward, upside down, horizontal or wrapped around a tree in his father's frustration. No matter what one does with it, a golf club is always a golf club.

Then, in the sixth year of his life, the child goes to school and is shown something that roughly resembles a golf club—the letter *d.* Only now he has to understand that if the letter is moved, it becomes a *b* or a *p* or a *q* or, if the handwriting is imprecise, an *h* or a *g*—all of which are different things. Similarly, a word is not always the same regardless of its position. *Saw*, reversed, becomes *was*. *Dog* becomes *god*, *cat* becomes *tac*, *rat* becomes *tar* and so on.

A child's preschool training hampers him in learning to read in another and more serious way. He has had relatively little experience with linear objects. He exists, prior to going to school, largely in a three-dimensional world of toys, balls and bats, knives and forks, water glasses, and other objects which have depth and shape he can touch. He has had relatively less experience with two-dimensional linear objects, which is what letters and numbers are. He is simply less accustomed to functioning and conceiving of a linear world.

Even the limited experience he has had in working with linear objects has not particularly prepared him to work with letters. He has colored, painted and drawn cats and dogs, people and other figures. With few exceptions, the letters in the English alphabet don't resemble cats and dogs and people. Letters consist of curved and straight lines in various combinations. Even the reading-readiness studies he has in kindergarten are not particularly helpful, for there he usually learns to differentiate between cat and pumpkin faces and other objects. It must be said that the preschool training of children might be more helpful if the child worked more with letter-like forms, rather than drawings of objects. It might help accustom him to the forms of letters that he will be using in learning to read in the first grade.

The initial task to be accomplished in learning to read is differentiating and identifying (not necessarily by name) the letters of the alphabet. This is a basic departure from the manner in which the child learned to speak. Although he differentiated between the sounds of English, he was not required to identify them. He didn't have to know that he was uttering a long *a* sound or a short *e* sound or any other, nor that the sound was part of his language. But in reading it is vital that he identify the letters, *even with the look-say method of reading*. He must discriminate at least the first and last letter of the word. When identifying the word *cat*, he is not required to identify the *c* and *t* by name, but he has to know that they are not *d* and *a* or other letters. He has to be able to distinguish the shapes of letters and discriminate them from others. In writing letters, the ability to discriminate is even more essential.

In neurological terms, the child, when he discriminates between letters (or the shapes of any objects), is using visual perception. The term *perception* is given a variety of different meanings by those who use it. The psychologist gives the term a broad meaning, to encompass anything a person becomes aware of in his environment. The dictionary defines *perception* as anything known of an object; the seeing or hearing of it; direct acquaintance with anything through the senses. Psychologists R. M. Mowbray and T. Ferguson Rodger[3] define *disordered perception* as the inability to organize stimuli in a meaningful fashion. *Stedman's Medical Dictionary* says perception is "the mental process by which the nature of an object is recognized through the association of a memory of its other qualities with the special sense, bringing it to consciousness."[4]

We use *perception* in a narrower sense—defining it as the ability to be aware of and conceive of a pattern or shape. This is a higher-order sensory function and involves interpretation and integration of the basic information of sight, hearing, touch, etc. In *visual perception* this is the recognition that a triangle, the end of a tent and a capital *A* are the same shape; in auditory perception, the recognition of a tune or melody played in a different key; and in touch, the ability to correctly identify by touch alone the textures of velvet and denim. In reading, *visual perception* means the ability to differentiate between the letters *d* and *b*, for example; *auditory perception* means the ability to differentiate between the sounds of the words *leaf* and *leave*.

Two major comments ought to be made about perception. First, it is difficult to know how a child fails to perceive. For example, if a child has a disorder of visual perception and he is asked to draw a triangle and renders it poorly so that it resembles an oval—does he do it because his brain is unaware that a triangle is composed of three straight lines connected by three angles? Or does his brain receive this information but is unaware of its significance, causing him to neglect this information? We don't know the answer.

Second, perception is learned. This has been shown by research with persons blind from birth who have regained their
sight through surgery. Psychologist D. O. Hebb has written a
fascinating account of this research[5]:

> The idea that one has to learn to see a triangle must sound
> extremely improbable, and so I shall now present the evidence
> to this effect more systematically. We have seen that the percep-
> tions of the congenitally blind after operation are almost com-
> pletely lacking in identity. Senden reports cases in which there
> was an immediate perception of differences in two figures seen
> together, but also one definite instance in which even this was not
> possible. Thus the patient sometimes saw differences between a
> sphere and cube, sometimes not. Color has been found to domi-
> nate form persistently in the first vision of these patients. Eleven
> months after operation the color names learned by a patient in
> hospital were retained, but the little that had been learned of form
> was forgotten. An egg, potato, and cube of sugar were seen by a
> patient repeatedly, until naming was prompt, but then were not
> recognized when put into colored light; the cube was well named
> when it was seen on the table or in the investigator's hand but not
> recognized when suspended by a thread with a change of back-
> ground.
>
> Such patients, when learning has proceeded far enough, mani-
> fest the characteristic generalizations of the normal person, so the
> initial difficulties are not to be put down to structural defects of
> the sensory apparatus.
>
> Riesen has fully confirmed the conclusion that ordinary visual
> perception in higher mammals presupposes a long learning period.
> His observations concerning the almost complete visual incapacity
> of chimpanzees reared in darkness, and the slowness of learning,
> are of the greatest importance. They show that Senden's similar re-
> sults with man are not due to some inadequacy of the clinical tests,
> nor peculiarly human.

Hebb then writes:

> The course of perceptal learning in man is gradual, proceeding
> from a dominance of color, through a period of separate attention
> to each part of a figure, to a gradually arrived at identification of
> the whole as a whole: an apparently simultaneous instead of a
> serial apprehension. A patient was trained to discriminate square
> from triangle over a period of 13 days, and had learned so little in

this time "that he could not report their form without counting corners one after another. . . . And yet it seems that the recognition process was beginning already to be automatic, so that some day the judgment 'square' would be given with simple vision, which would then easily lead to the belief that form was always simultaneously given" [Hebb is quoting Senden]. The shortest time in which a patient approximated to normal perception, even when learning was confined to a small number of objects, seems to have been about a month.

It is possible then that the normal human infant goes through the same process, and that we are able to see a square as such in a single glance only as the result of complex learning. The notion seems unlikely, because of the utter simplicity of such a perception to the normal adult. But no such argument can be valid, since Lashley has shown that subjective simplicity and immediacy may be very deceptive as an index of physiological simplicity. There are moreover residual traces of learning in normal perception, and hints of its complexity.

Gellerman reports that chimpanzees and two-year-old children recognized a triangle that had been rotated through 120° from the training position, but (in the one protocol that is given) responded selectively only *after* a head rotation; and persistent head rotation continued in the later discriminations. Older human subjects do not need to make the same receptor adjustment to recognize the figure in two positions, and so this generalization may be a learned capacity, simple as it seems to us.

This research into the nature of perceptual learning, which Hebb has summarized so well, is of the greatest importance in the teaching of reading. The distinctive shapes of letters and numbers do not leap into recognition as they do with an adult. The child must examine the figures to detect their distinguishing characteristics. For example, when identifying a square, he actually counts the corners.

This was shown by an experiment related by Hebb,[6] as follows:

The subject is shown a diagram such as

x	e	a	q
r	l	i	s
o	f	z	g
d	y	u	p

and studies it until he has, apparently, an image of the whole square and can "look at" it and read the letters off, one by one. If he really has such an image, it will not matter in what direction he is asked to "read." Actually, it is found that the subject cannot reproduce the letters as fast from right to left as from left to right, or promptly give the four letters, *p, z, l, x,* that make up the diagonal from lower right to upper left. So what seems a simple, immediately given image of the whole is actually a serial reconstruction of parts of the figure. An "image" of triangle or square is simpler, longer practiced, but may be fundamentally the same. The perception of such figures also may involve a temporal sequence.

Thus, the normal child must *learn* to discriminate the shapes of letters, whether he is being taught by a phonic or a look-say method.

IDENTIFYING LETTERS

At this point it is proper to consider the difficulty which the normal child has in identifying letters. The Cornell study sought to discover how a child differentiates one letter from another.

It was obvious to the Cornell scientists that letters of the alphabet could not be used to discover how the child learns them. The children being tested might know one or several letters. They would at least have a familiarity with them. To avoid this difficulty, the researchers prepared a group of letter-like forms consisting of straight and curved lines such as those used in letters. Then, 12 variants were prepared of each standard letter-like form. In some of the variants the forms were rotated or reversed (as letters are); or curved lines were used instead of straight ones; or there were breaks in the lines that did not exist in the standard form; or there were perspective transformations in which the standard figure was slanted backward or forward.

Then the Cornell psychologists asked a group of children, ages four through eight, to pick out copies of the standard form from a group that included all of its transformations. The youngsters were to select only the exact copies of the standard form. The errors made by the children were scored and the errors classified according to the type of transformation.

Results of the test showed that the visual discrimination of children improved from ages four to eight, but that some discriminations between forms were harder to make than others and that improvement in discrimination varies from form to form. For example, errors for perspective transformations were very numerous among four-year-olds and still numerous among eight-year-olds. This was not considered critical because English letters do not normally contain perspectives, that is, the letters are all made to appear flat. At least in the primary grades, there is no attempt to give the letters the appearance of depth.

Of greater significance were these results: changes of break or close, such as between a *c* and an *o*, are easiest for children. Even the youngest tested made relatively few errors and none of the eight-year-olds made a mistake.

Errors for rotations and reversals—*d* and *b*, *p* and *q*, *M* and *W*, *c* and *u*—were very high among the four-year-olds, but dropped to nearly zero by age eight.

Errors for changes from line to curve—*v* and *u*, for example—were relatively numerous (depending on the number of changes) among the youngest children but showed a rapid drop among the older ones, almost to zero for the eight-year-olds.

The Cornell researchers then tried the same transformations of real letters on the five-year-old group and found that the same confusions resulted. This indicated that problems in discrimination apply generally and not just to the specific forms drawn for the experiment.

Some comments can be made concerning the results of this experiment. First, a child's ability to distinguish one letter from another improves with age. By age eight he is an expert, making hardly any mistakes at all. But the child of eight is usually in the third grade. What of the first-grader who is having trouble discriminating one letter from another? Is he receiving proper help from his teacher? Teachers work quite hard on reversals and rotations, but do they realize that line-to-curve distinctions also cause difficulty? The answer to these questions is somewhat important, for the Cornell study showed that at age six the children tested made about 18 percent errors in rotation and reversal and 26 percent in line-to-curve transformations.

How does a child differentiate one letter from another? If the answer to this question could be obtained, it would open a new avenue of teaching, in which instruction can be given to the child to help him distinguish one letter from another, thus eliminating some of the time-consuming trial and error of self-discovery.*

The Cornell experimenters formed two hypotheses concerning how children might discriminate letters. In one it was assumed that the child builds up a kind of model of each letter and then compares until he makes a match, or, in the other, that he discovers how letters differ and recognizes them by distinctive features.

To test which hypothesis was correct, the psychologists worked with a group of kindergarten children, training them to discriminate between letter-like forms similar to those used in the earlier experiment. Then the children were divided into three groups. Group one was given new forms to learn, forms which varied in new ways from the same standards of discrimination they had already learned. Group two was given new sets of forms which differed in the same ways as the forms they had already learned. The third group was a control given both new standards and new dimensions of difference to discriminate.

---

* The use—he would say abuse—of self-discovery learning in reading instruction has been criticized by psychologist Roger Brown in an article "A Dispute about Reading" in the book *Human Learning in the School*,[7] as follows:

"The need for phonetic attack on new words is generally recognized by educators of the look-and-say persuasion, but for one reason or another they believe the necessary generalizations should be incidentally learned or, if directly taught, postponed until the second or third grade. What are the reasons for this belief? Dolch and Bloomster have said: 'It is true that the use of phonics means the use of generalizations, *that generalizations are best learned inductively*, and that sight words are the basis of inductive reasoning.' (Italics my own.) The italicized portion of this sentence is hardly a common-sense observation. Why does the scientist write out his laws, the chef his recipes, the professional golfer his instructions for the novice, if not to spare the rest of us inductive labor? We benefit from the experiences of our predecessors by reading the generalizations reformed. It may be that the Darwinian Theory of Evolution is best learned inductively—best in the sense of most unforgettably. But if it had to be learned that way, most of us would live without a theory of evolution. On the face of it, a generalization is more rapidly and certainly learned when it is explicitly stated. In addition, there are experimental results to show that incidental learning is slow and uncertain by comparison with directed learning. The educator, who would claim that phonetic generalizations are better learned by incidental induction than by direct formulation with examples, assumes the burden of proof. His claim does not conform to popular belief, nor has it been demonstrated in the laboratory. If you really want your pupil to learn a phonetic rule, it seems sensible to tell him the rule."

It was inferred that better performance by the first group would suggest that discrimination learning proceeded by construction of a model of the standards against which the variants could be matched. If the second group performed better it would suggest that distinctive differences had been detected by the children.

Results showed that both groups one and two performed better than the control group, and that group two performed best, making 39 errors to group one's 69. "We infer from these results," Dr. Eleanor Gibson wrote in *Science,* "that, while children probably do learn prototypes of letter shapes, the prototypes themselves are not the original basis for differentiation. The most relevant kind of training for discrimination is practice which provides experience with the characteristic differences that distinguish the set of items. Features which are actually distinctive for letters could be emphasized by presenting letters in contrast pairs."[8]

The experimenters made an effort, unfortunately not completed, to determine which features a child distinguishes. It seemed to indicate that children distinguish between curved and straight lines and between the obliqueness of a line, as in *A, K, N,* and *Z.* It is to be hoped these experiments can be continued until it is known precisely which features of letters help a child distinguish it from another.*

The Cornell study seems to indicate that a teacher would be wise to drill students on discriminating between letters as well as identifying them.

---

* We would like to suggest that some experimenters develop what might be called an *Initial Perceptual Alphabet* (IPA), a concept similar to the *Initial Teaching Alphabet* (ITA) which was discussed on page 24. ITA, it will be remembered, is an attempt to circumvent the phonic irregularities of the English alphabet by creating letter figures for each of the common phonic elements in the language, 44 in all, so that each ITA letter represents one English sound. After learning by this method, the child later transfers easily to a regular alphabet. We consider this a most appealing addition to the theory of reading instruction. We are suggesting that a similar technique be used to circumvent some of the visual confusions in the alphabet, such as the *b* and *d, p* and *q, m* and *w, u* and *v.* If another form were substituted for one of the confusing letters—there is no reason that squares, triangles and other geometric forms cannot be used—it would simplify the visual aspect of reading as the ITA alphabet does the auditory aspect. The child, after benefiting from his IPA exposure, could then be transferred to the regular letter forms.

READING AND WRITING ARE RELATED

Another team of psychologists at Cornell sought to determine the correlation between reading and writing. The hypothesis was stated well by the researchers, James J. Gibson and Harry Osser:

> In the acquisition of language it is clear that a child never learns to understand speech without at the same time learning to speak. The circularity of speaking and hearing has always been recognized and the degree to which the auditory feedback controls the process of uttering words has recently been studied experimentally. What has not been so clear is that a child never learns to *read* without at the same time learning to *write*. Reading and writing are different terms and often seem to be thought of as different school subjects. Nevertheless, the visual feedback which controls the manual art of writing is quite analogous to the auditory feedback which controls the vocal art of speaking. Just as one cannot speak without hearing one's speech, so one cannot write without, in a peculiar sense, reading one's writing.

Gibson and Osser pointed out that what a child must learn in order to read and write is that "speech sounds can appear, and can be *made* to appear on a visible surface."

Is it useful in the classroom to have the child write letters as a means of helping him to discriminate and identify them? Gibson and Osser sought to discover this by having 20 children, four to six years of age, punch out letters on a typewriter. Some of the children used a typewriter that contained a ribbon, thus permitting them to see the letters they made. The remainder used typewriters without ribbons and thus received no visual reinforcement of their efforts.

Results showed that those children who used typewriters with ribbons performed significantly better than those who merely punched a typewriter key. The results are interesting in that they showed that merely by looking at letters the child made with a typewriter helped his discrimination of them. It is unfortunate, however, that typewriters were used in this experiment. If another group of children had written or printed the letters by hand, it is likely that they would have shown even greater reinforcement of their ability to discriminate. There is abundant evidence that tactile perception provides an avenue of learning. Helen Keller used this method exclusively. Schools experimenting with the teaching of dyslexic children with severe visual and auditory imperception are obtaining good results by teaching children to read by means of tactile perception, that is, having them feel letters and write them in sandboxes or on blackboards. (Grace Fernald[9] has done the most significant investigation of the efficacy of tactile methods of teaching reading.)

We believe there is great value in teaching reading and writing simultaneously, rather than as separate subjects in the curriculum. Writing the letters aids the child in distinguishing and identifying them. He is using visual perception when he sees the letters, auditory perception when the teacher speaks them, and tactile perception when he writes them on paper or the blackboard. The normal child thus is using three broad avenues to language comprehension. This three-pronged learning process is of value even after he has learned the first step in reading and can distinguish and identify letters. Writing, as well as seeing and hearing, help him to learn the spelling patterns and then the sentence structures which are characteristic of English. In short, writing is a most valuable tool in the teaching of reading.

IDENTIFYING WORDS

The importance of teaching children to discriminate one letter from another very early in the instructional program was illustrated in another Cornell experiment. Performed by Gabrielle Edelman, this investigation produced results which have far-reaching significance for the practicing classroom teacher.

Miss Edelman sought to discover the cues by which a nonreader or beginning reader identifies a word he has never seen, whether the same cues are used to recognize a long word and a short word, whether nonreaders and beginning readers use the same cues, and whether boys and girls use the same cues. Two groups were selected; 50 kindergarteners and 50 first-graders, each chosen at random from public schools and each divided equally among boys and girls.

The children were shown a card on which was printed a nonsense word, for example, *cug*. Then the youngsters were shown response cards in randon arrangement. They were to point to the word on one of the response cards which was identical or most resembled the word they had seen on the first card. The response cards were arranged so as to determine (1) whether the children cued on the basis of shape by selecting *arp,* which has the same shape as *cug* but all the letters changed; (2) by the first letter by selecting *che,* which has the same first letter as *cug* but different second and third letters and the shape changed; (3) on the basis of the second letter by selecting *tuk,* which has the same second letter as *cug* but the first and third letters and the shape are different; or (4) on the basis of the final letter by selecting *ilg,* which has the same third letter but the first two and the shape are changed. A similar system was worked out for five-letter nonsense words. In both the three-letter and the five-letter tests, the response cards were presented in varying order so no cue could be based on sequence. There were eight combinations of each three-letter word and 52 combinations of each five-letter word.

The results were different depending on the size of the word and, surprisingly, on the sex of the participants. The first letter of both the long- and short-word forms was the cue most utilized by nonreaders (kindergarteners) and beginning readers (first-graders). The last letter is also an important cue, especially for kindergarteners, and more so in short words than in long ones. Boys tend to recognize words on the basis of the first more than the last letter. Girls, while using both first and last, place greater emphasis on the second letter than boys do, as shown by the following table:

			Five-Letter Words			
Cues:	SHAPE	FIRST	SECOND	THIRD	FOURTH	FIFTH
Kindergarten	330	1673	540	755	518	1365
1st Grade	80	2497	757	693	287	930
Boys	214	1886	589	780	445	1208
Girls	196	2284	708	614	360	1087

(The figures represent the number of times children recognized words on the basis of certain cues.)

Gabrielle Edelman concluded from her experiment that "theories which propose that nonreaders and/or beginning readers recognize words as wholes by their shape have not been supported in this study. The shapes of words, offered as a cue next to letter cues, was rejected in favor of letter cues . . . in this experiment." She pointed out that the study showed that the first letter is the most important cue in whole-word recognition and that the last letter is next in importance. She theorized that this phenomenon may lie in the primacy of the first letter and the recency of the last, or simply that the first and last letters, since they are bordered on one side by white space, stand out more than those letters embedded in the middle of a word.

> The major implication for the teaching of reading [according to Miss Edelman, a view which we share] is that the basic belief on which the whole-word method of teaching reading lies (i.e., the belief that children recognize words by their shape) is incorrect. Educators may believe the child is attending to the whole word, when he is actually utilizing certain letter cues. Helping pupils learn the letters well so that they may use letter cues to the best of their ability would be an important teaching improvement.

This information about the manner in which a normal child recognizes and identifies the graphic symbols on a page is of the greatest possible importance in teaching of reading. It offers, we believe, some insights into the problems of the normal child in learning to read and to some ways teachers can assist this child over these hurdles.

But our primary purpose in including this material in this book is to show the monstrous task that confronts the dyslexic child with poor visual perception. If he does not correctly perceive the shape of the letter *d*, for example, just try to imagine his difficulty in differentiating the letter from a *b*, *p* or *q*. If he does not correctly perceive the shape of an *m*, how can he distinguish it from a *w?* And making such distinctions is the absolutely essential first step in reading. This child, even if his impairment is a mild one, needs a great deal of time-consuming help in surmounting the first step in reading.

6.

Translating the Marks to Sound

THE SECOND STEP in learning to read is for the child to decode letters into sound. How does the child accomplish this? Eleanor Gibson discussed the possible methods quite lucidly in her *Science* article[1]:

> This [decoding] process, common sense as many psychologists would tell us, is simply a matter of associating a graphic stimulus [letter] with the appropriate spoken response—that is to say, it is the traditional stimulus-response paradigm, a kind of paired-associate learning.
>
> Obvious as this description seems, problems arise when one takes a closer look. Here are just a few. The graphic code is related to the speech code by rules of correspondence. If these rules are known, decoding of new items is predictable. Do we want to build up, one by one, automatically cued responses, or do we want to teach with transfer [to new letters and words] in mind? If we want to teach for transfer, how do we do it? Should the child be aware that this is a code game with rules? Or will induction of rules be automatic? What units of both codes should we start with? Should we start with single letters, in the hope that knowledge of single-letter-to-sound relationships will yield the most transfer? Or should we start with whole words, in the hope that component relationships will be induced?

PHONIC VERSUS LOOK-SAY METHOD

An experiment was established to determine whether the phonic or look-say method is best in teaching a child to learn *new* words. Carol Bishop[2] performed the experiment, which produced rather surprising results.

Mrs. Bishop simulated the child's process of learning to read by teaching adults to read Arabic words which had no meaning to them. Thus there could be no association by meaning. Only the sound and visual aspects of the letters and words could be used.

To begin the experiment 12 Arabic characters, each with a one-to-one letter-sound correspondence, were selected. There were eight consonants and four vowels combined to form two sets of words. A native speaker of the language recorded the 12 letter-sounds and two sets of words on tape, and each letter and word was printed on a card.

The subjects to be tested, all college students, were divided into three groups, all of whom learned to pronounce the sets of words by listening to the recording and repeating the words. In the second stage, group one listened to and repeated the 12 letter-sounds and then learned to associate the letters with the sounds. This was a phonic approach. The second group set out to learn the eight Arabic words rather than the individual letters. This was the look-say method. The third or control group spent its time on an unrelated task.

Finally, in the third stage of the experiment, all the subjects learned to read the set of words they had heard in stage one, responding to the presentation of the words on a card by pronouncing it. All the subjects were tested on their ability to give correct letter-sound following the presentation of each printed letter and they were asked to explain how they tried to learn the words.

The phonic group performed best, learning all eight words in seven trials, indicating that phonics training makes it easier for a person to learn new words. Those trained in the look-say method needed 15 trials to learn the new words. The control group did quite poorly, requiring 25 trials.

Carol Bishop also tested the subjects on the number of letter-sound correspondences they had learned. The phonic group, on the average, knew a greater number of sounds that the letters make than the look-say group, but, startlingly, 12 of the 20 adults in the look-say group, 60 percent of its members, had learned all 12 letter-sound correspondences *without any training*. The other eight members of the look-say group who did not use letter-sound correspondences performed no better on this task than the control subjects.

This is not a perfect experiment. Unfortunately, it used adults instead of children. The adults may have had some previous exposure to phonics in English. They are certainly more able to figure out that the sounds the letters make is important in learning new words than six-year-old children are. Also, the experiment involved only single-letter to single-sound correspondences, leaving questions unanswered about how more complex letter-to-sound correspondences would work.

Despite these flaws, this experiment is the best evidence available to date that (1) phonics provides the best method of learning *new* words, and (2) that many individuals who are taught the look-say method teach themselves the phonic method. What is disconcerting in this experiment is that eight, or 40 percent, of the adult subjects taught the look-say method failed to teach themselves phonics so as to learn the sounds made by the individual letters in the words they learned to read.

This experiment certainly indicates, at least, an explanation for some phenomena long observed in the teaching of reading. One can begin to understand why a high percentage of children learn to read regardless of the method they are taught. If taught phonics, a majority of the children teach themselves to recognize whole words. If taught the look-say method, they teach themselves enough phonics to learn to sound out new words. But, because a significant segment of the children who are taught the look-say method fail to teach themselves phonics, it would seem that educators have been wise to provide them with some training in phonics.

PHONIC IRREGULARITIES

Training in phonics certainly has a role in learning to read, but what role? Several of the Cornell experiments go a long way toward answering this question which has puzzled educators for some time.

Dr. Harry Levin performed experiments which tackled head-on the problem of phonic irregularities. As is commonly observed, one of the difficulties with phonics is that English is full of contradictions. For example, a child may be taught that *a* makes the short sound as in "r*a*t." Then the child is confronted with the long *a* sound as in "r*a*te." So, the child is taught a spelling rule that when the letter (not the sound) *e* is added to the word it makes the vowel "say its name." But the child quickly discovers this rule does not apply to the *a* in "m*a*y"—there is no *e* to make the vowel say its name—or "c*a*re," which has an *e* and a short vowel. The obvious difficulties a child can have with these confusions led celebrated linguist Leonard Bloomfield[3] to suggest that beginning reading materials should be carefully selected to teach only phonic regularities, leaving the irregularities to be introduced gradually later.

Dr. Levin sought to determine by experimentation whether Bloomfield is correct. He gave one group of first-graders a list of simple words to learn that were highly regular phonetically and followed it by a list that was irregular. A second group was given two lists, both of which were irregular. Results showed that the group that became accustomed to irregularities from the outset performed better than the group that started with regularities and then went to irregularities, thus indicating that teachers are better off to tackle the problem of phonic irregularities at the beginning of instruction.

The Cornell experiments further indicate that instruction of phonics is more valuable in the early stages of instruction, rather than later as some authorities have recommended. Psychologist Roger Brown is of the same opinion:[4]

> Some educators think it best to teach phonetics directly, but argue that such training ought not to be used before the second grade. Until that time, it has been claimed, children have insufficient mental maturity to make use of abstract phonetic principles. Dolch and Bloomster found that first-grade children taught a look-and-say method fail to form phonetic generalizations which they could use in attacking new words. The authors conclude that a mental age of seven years, with usually a second-grade standing, must be attained before a child can benefit from phonic training, and that all such training ought to be postponed until he has reached that age. Quite obviously their results did not demonstrate that first-grade children are unable to benefit from phonic training since the children of this study were not given *explicit*

phonic training. First-grade children know the rules of games that are fully as complicated as the rules involved in spelling. Furthermore, they are rather accomplished speakers of English, which means they have formed many concepts and learned complicated grammatical conventions. It seems unlikely that spelling rules are beyond them.

THE BASIC READING UNIT

The importance of early phonic training was shown in Cornell experiments which sought to determine what "the critical unit of language" is in reading. Does a child learn to read word by word, syllable by syllable, letter by letter?

He definitely does not do the last. Experiments have shown that when a person is shown letters tachistoscopically—that is, one after the other in sequence for a measured period of time— he reads with only the greatest difficulty. If he sees each letter for only 100 milliseconds, he can read words of six letters with only 20 percent accuracy. If given 375 milliseconds to view each letter, his probability of accuracy is still under 100 percent—and he has had over two seconds to look at each word. Said Eleanor Gibson: "We can conclude that however graphemes* are processed perceptually in reading, it is not a letter-by-letter sequence of acts."[5]

What are the smallest units a person reads? Dr. Gibson said, as a result of her studies, "It is my belief that the smallest component units in written English are spelling patterns. By a spelling pattern, I mean a cluster of graphemes in a given environment which has an invariant pronunciation according to the rules of English." An experienced reader of English is quite familiar with these rules, although he may not have verbalized them. For example, a *q* is without exception followed by a *u;* the *ck* combination is common, but it almost always appears at the end of a word; English words frequently begin with graphemes such as *br, cr, pr, wh, th, ch, sh, st,* and many more, but those combinations of letters are rarely if ever reversed; common endings of words are *ion, ing, es, ed, ist, ish, est, ich, ent* and many more, but again the order of letters is seldom, if ever,

---

* A letter or a basic group of letters, such as *gr, cr, th,* is called a "grapheme" when written, and a "phoneme" when uttered.

reversed or otherwise altered; when two vowels occur together, *i* precedes *e* except after *c* or in certain other exceptions, *o* precedes *a, i* frequently goes before *a, e* before *a, o* before *u*, along with several others that occur regularly and with few exceptions.

An exhaustive list of English spelling rules would be quite long.* An experienced reader becomes unconsciously adept at these rules, but the key both to the rules and to using them is that the spelling patterns have an invariant relationship to *sound* patterns. *Ith* says itself, so does *ese, ing, gra, pro, ich* and all the rest. The experienced reader, then, uses spelling-to-sound correspondence.

The importance of spelling patterns might be illustrated with typing. The beginning typist starts out typing each letter individually, but with practice develops speed by typing in familiar combinations of letters. The fingers become accustomed (in reality, brain pathways are established) for all of the familiar English spelling. The typist types in syllables and whole words that become familiar from long practice, needing to type letter-by-letter only those words which are long, unfamiliar or which defy conventional spelling.

Spelling patterns of English have a parallel in syntax. The conventional order of sentence structure is subject, verb, predicate. If the verb precedes the subject, we are accustomed to expect the sentence to be a question. We have a vast repertoire of rules governing the content and sequence of phrases and clauses inserted in a sentence. The essence of lucidness, whether in speech or writing, is that these rules of syntax are followed, for we are trained almost from birth to expect the words in our native language to follow patterns in accordance with rules prescribed by long usage. The experienced reader makes constant use of these regular patterns of sentence structure.

Thus, he obtains meaning from the whole context of what he has read and is reading. If he has been reading in the past tense, he expects a continuation of the past tense, unless there is a chronological progression in time toward the present or future, or tense is changed for particular emphasis. He tends, also, to pay particular attention to those words which provide the meaning to a sentence. For example: Bring me a ————. To the experienced

---

* And such a list has never been prepared!

reader, whatever word or words go in the blank (glass of water, book, chair, etc.) gives the sentence its essential meaning. He reads all the words, to be sure. He knows the words were *bring* and not *give, me* and not *him, a* and not *the* (particular) chair or book. In short, he gathered the meaning of the entire sentence by reading words that followed rules of spelling-to-sound correspondence and that were arranged in sequences in accordance with accustomed rules of grammar and syntax.

THE IMPORTANCE OF SPELLING

If this is what the experienced reader does, what does the beginning reader do? Cornell experimenters Eleanor Gibson, Anne Pick, Harry Osser and Marcia Hammond made these comments on this question:

> A child who learns to read (well) is forming useful spelling-to-sound habits based on these rules, whether he could tell you so or not. Even if he is taught by some method which makes it difficult, he must eventually discover the important spelling-to-sound correlations, if he is to be able to generate for himself the way to read new words.
>
> From this starting position, we can proceed to the statement of a psychological hypothesis which has some testable consequences. Reading consists of decoding graphic material to the phonemic patterns of spoken language which have already been mastered when reading is begun. The units to be decoded are not single letters, for these have no invariant acoustic match in our language. The whole word is possible, but is uneconomical as a training unit for it provides no basis for independent decoding of new graphic combinations. The hypothesis advanced is that the reading task is essentially that of discovering higher-order invariants, the spelling-to-sound correlations. . . .
>
> It is assumed that the individual discovers these grapheme-phoneme correspondences as he learns to read, even if he is not specifically taught them. He may not be able to draw up a set of rules but he "has" them, if he is a good reader, just as a young child "has" grammar long before he can formulate rules for it. Once he has them, any letter-combinations which follow the rules are functional units.

To test this hypothesis, the experimenters formed a list of nonsense words which were pronounceable according to the rules of English and a second list of nonsense words, consisting of the same letters, which were unpronounceable or extremely difficult to pronounce. Thus *dink* was pronounceable and *nkid* was not; *glox* and *xogl; lods* and *dsol; besks* and *skseb; brelp* and *lpebr; blasps* and *spsabl; glurck* and *ckurgl.* The words were projected on a screen and college students were asked to write them down. The pronounceable words were perceived consistently and significantly more often. Said the experimenters:

> The results of this experiment demonstrate that a letter-group with a high spelling-to-sound correlation is reproduced more accurately than an equivalent letter-group with a low spelling-to-sound correlation. This result cannot be caused by a difference in the familiarity of the letters taken alone, or even the vowel- and consonant-clusters taken alone, for the same clusters were used in the two lists. It must be due to the existence of higher-order graphic units: the letter-combinations of English writing that function as relatively stable units in grapheme-phoneme correspondence.
>
> Practically, this result suggests strongly that the proper unit for analyzing the process of reading (and writing) is not the alphabetical letter but the spelling pattern which has an invariant relationship with a phonemic pattern. This may be of great importance for children's learning to read and write.

How early in the instructional process does the beginning reader start to detect spelling-to-sound correspondences? To determine this, the Cornell researchers designed an experiment to compare children at the end of the first grade and at the end of the third grade to test their ability to recognize familiar three-letter words. (It would be assumed that the first-graders had not yet had phonics training, while the third-graders had.)

The words were taken from a first-grade reading list and arranged into meaningless but pronounceable ones, and meaningless and unpronounceable ones. For example, *ran, nar, rna.* The words were shown tachistoscopically (each unit alone for a measured amount of time) to the children, who were required to spell them orally. The first-graders spelled out or read most accurately the familiar three-letter words (*ran*), but read the pronounceable combinations (*nar*) significantly better than the unpronounceable ones (*rna*). The third-grade children read all three-letter combinations with high and about equal accuracy. Both groups were also given some longer, nonsense words (*glurck* and *ckurgl*). The first-graders did poorly on these, but the third-graders were able to perceive the pronounceable pseudo words more often than the unpronounceable ones. Concludes Eleanor Gibson[6]:

> These results suggest that a child in the first stages of reading skill typically reads in short units, but has already generalized certain regularities of spelling-to-sound correspondence, so that three-letter pseudo words which fit the rules are more easily read as units. As skill develops, span increases, and a smaller difference can be observed for longer items. The longer items involve more complex conditional rules and longer clusters, so that the generalization must increase in complexity. The fact that a child can begin very early to perceive regularities of correspondence between the printed and spoken patterns, and transfer them to the reading of unfamiliar times as units, suggest that the opportunities for discovering the correspondences between patterns might well be enhanced in programming reading materials.

We would go a step further here and suggest to teachers that they consider the wisdom of actually instructing beginning readers in spelling-to-sound correspondence, rather than letting them figure them out by induction. (Roger Brown's simile of teaching Darwin's theory of evolution rather than letting each child figure it out for himself, which was quoted in Chapter 5, is most apropos here.) We hope that in the near future teachers will conduct experiments to determine the efficacy of instructing children in rules of spelling so as to speed their use of them in reading.

We further submit that, in reality, the development of spelling-to-sound correspondences as the "critical unit" in reading is but a variation—an important variation, to be sure—of the look-say method. The child learns to look, not at a whole word, perhaps, but at a spelling pattern and to say it. Learning spelling patterns involves sounding out words. The child must have some phonics, either teacher-taught or self-taught, if he is to learn the sounds conventional spellings make. But relatively soon, he begins to use a whole-word method. He uses the phonics to sound out the new words. He may sound it out several times until he becomes familiar with it. Then the process of familiarity amounts to looking at the word and saying what it is. His vocabulary of familiar words increases rapidly as he continues to read. His knowledge of familiar patterns and the rules of spelling and syntax enlarge. His ability to sound out words phonically becomes virtually automatic. The sight of the word as a whole triggers the sound and thus its meaning to him.

The research at Cornell and elsewhere seems to indicate—and as nonexperts in education we do not wish to be dogmatic about this—that most school instruction in reading has been sequentially backwards. These investigations seem to indicate that phonics should be taught first, not in the second grade; that very early spelling-to-sound correspondences should be pointed out; and that the whole-word method, based on spelling patterns rather than on the configuration of the word (which the child doesn't grasp anyhow), should come next.

READING FOR MEANING

The meaning of the words, which has been the major concern of a whole generation of American teachers, has a role in this hypothetical reading program, as was demonstrated by a fascinating experiment performed at Cornell by Eleanor Gibson, Carol Bishop, William Schiff and Jesse Smith. In this experiment, the researchers made up three letter trigrams. One type was unpronounceable and had no meaning. A second set was unpronounceable but had meaning. The third was pronounceable but had no meaning. Adults were tested to see which type of trigram was learned the easiest. Some of the trigrams were as follows:

Unpronounceable, no meaning	Unpronounceable, meaning	Pronounceable, no meaning
OKR	RKO	KOR
AVT	TVA	TAV
MBI	IBM	MIB
IFB	FBI	BIF
ACB	ABC	BAC
OTK	TKO	TOK
YNU	NYU	YUN
LFA	AFL	FAL

The study showed that pronounceable trigrams were easiest to learn (those in the third column), the meaningful ones next easiest, and unpronounceable, meaningless ones hardest. Thus, being able to pronounce a word, that is, sound it out, makes it easier to learn. The adults were subsequently tested on their ability to recall these trigrams. It was discovered that they were better able to recall those trigrams which had meaning, rather than those which were pronounceable or unpronounceable without meaning.

The conclusions from this experiment are that pronounceability is important to reading but that meaning is the key to remembering. The experimenters' discussion of this is of some value. They said (italics theirs):

> In the perception of *written* language, the perceiver must code the stimulus material into units of *spoken* language—that is first and foremost the reading task. But we do not speak in letters; we speak in syllables, words and larger functional units. A letter name is itself a morpheme, not an element of a speech unit. Since the reader must code the written letters into functional speech units, pronounceable letter combinations will obviously facilitate his task. But the kind of meaning present in IBM creates three units for reading rather than one. In the recognition and recall tasks, on the other hand, the stimulus items have already been read (coded into speech units). The task now is to hang onto them—store them for future "retrieval." . . . The category of pronounceable trigrams (if it could be called a category at all) is so large as to be of small help in retrieval. In other words, pronounceability is of the utmost help in structuring a unit—grouping the letters into a single item—but it is of little help in grouping those items under a single address. . . . On the other hand, the class of "well-known initials" does provide a common category for grouping items in storage. It provides a coding principle for retention.

Pronounceability is the key to reading, but meaning of the words is the limb from which recall hangs. In categorizing information which he has acquired and wishes to store for later recall, a child (or an adult) uses the meaning of the word rather than the pronounceability of it.

It is our belief that in the first three grades the major emphasis should be on teaching a child to read—translate a mark on paper into sound. The words which he sounds out or pronounces will be simple words and have meaning for him. Emphasis on meaning in these grades, with the exception just noted, is not well placed.*

But in the upper primary grades, we believe an important change occurs. At some point in the fourth, fifth or sixth grade, the child develops a larger reading vocabulary than an auditory one. He begins to learn new words through reading. He has the ability to sound out and pronounce words the meaning of which he doesn't know. He now turns to the dictionary (or other sources) to discover the meaning. It is at this point—not in the first grade, it seems to us—that emphasis on silent reading for meaning makes the most sense, for the child now reads to learn where formerly he was learning to read.**

The aim of reading instruction is to have every child reach this point where he reads for meaning. After that the child teaches himself, improving his reading vocabulary with almost every item he reads. We believe, too, that there might be value in drilling the fifth- and sixth-grader in the look-say method (perhaps using flash cards) so as to increase the speed and efficiency with which he recognizes those common words which are the basis of our language.

WRITING AND SPELLING

Handwriting (or printing) is to reading as speaking is to hearing—it follows as the motor application of a sensory function. A child reads before he writes—or learns to read faster than he learns to write—because writing is an additional function. Writing is a double code (mark on paper to sound to meaning) with the addition of motor coordination. A child learns to read through writing. He uses a visual control and a tactile control

* The child who reads but cannot comprehend should be studied because he may be retarded, may be preoccupied with emotional problems or worries, may be culturally deprived, or may be such a marginal reader that he is forced to ignore the meaning. The latter can be tested in all but the beginning reader by having him read quite simple material for meaning.

** It should be pointed out that the Waysiders may never get to this point, and psychologists may observe a tailing off of verbal IQ. The child is not learning by reading. He is not obtaining information as normal children do, and is falling behind his contemporaries informationally and intellectually.

and a position control as feedbacks to the brain from his hand. Handwriting improves his reading and reinforces his visual perception, and this works in the normal child as well as the child with perceptual difficulties. Reading and writing should be taught simultaneously or in close proximity.

An aspect of writing instruction that seems to bother teachers is that the child is often so very sloppy. This is so more frequently with boys than girls. The causes of the lack of graphic neatness in boys are not fully known. There may be some neurological basis for it in the slower development of the fine motor coordination needed for precise handwriting. Another factor certainly is that boys are less motivated to be neat than girls. Being able to color between the lines* or produce a neat paper is not a particular status symbol for most boys. In any event, it is possible for teachers to make too much of students' lack of neatness. Forming printed or cursive letters legibly is important, but in this era of the typewriter and dictating machine, it is far from vital. In another era when all records were kept by hand, legible, even artistic handwriting was vital. Today it is far from necessary. Indeed, cursive writing seems to be disappearing. Where is it used in business, science or the professions?

Spelling is another school subject closely allied to reading. It should be said here that there is a neurological disorder of spelling (writing words)—*dysgraphia*. This disability is commonly seen with dyslexia, as a reflection of the reading disorder; but a pure dysgraphic, the child who can read but cannot spell (write words) for neurological reasons, is seen less frequently.

For most children, spelling reflects the method by which a child was taught to read. If the child was taught by the look-say method and did not figure out for himself the letter-to-sound and spelling-to-sound correspondences, he is apt to be a poorer speller than the child blessed with teacher-taught or self-taught phonics. A child can be a good reader and a poor speller or vice versa as a reflection of the way he was taught to read. But there can be many individual variations. In general it may be said that

* We doubt that using coloring of pictures as a tool to teach coordination works very well. As drawing and identifying pumpkin and cat's faces is not ideal preparation for reading, so coloring is not the best preparation for writing. We suspect that drawing and identifying letter-like forms is a more useful readiness tool in kindergarten.

the child who isn't even close in his spelling may have a neurological disorder, while the child who makes minor misselections of letters probably lacks training in phonic and spelling rules.

We believe that teachers might consider the wisdom of formally presenting at least the common rules of spelling. Some of this is done, but perhaps there is need for more extensive exposition of spelling rules. The advantages in allowing the child to figure this out for himself seem difficult to appreciate.

In the last several chapters we have presented a body of information that seems pertinent to the reading process in the normal child. Our primary purpose in this has been to set the stage for understanding how neurological disorders can inhibit the reading process. If a child has impaired visual perception, for example, he can have difficulty in the first task in reading, discriminating the shapes of letters. Auditory imperception can make training in phonics quite unproductive. There are other illustrations which we will develop fully later.

We believe, however, that this material which we have presented may compose some of the ingredients for a new approach to reading instruction. These research findings and other pieces of information are hardly definitive. They scarcely qualify as a blueprint for a new method of teaching reading. But it is our hope that teachers and educators will feel this information has sufficient merit to warrant further investigation that might lead to improved reading instruction. We feel reading instruction is the effort of a triumvirate—the psychologist, the educator and the physician. The psychologists have made a major contribution with their experiments. The information which will follow will reveal much about the neurological abnormalities. The task of educators now, it seems to us, is to take this information and apply it to practical classroom usage.

To summarize, we believe educators should conduct investigations to determine the practical efficacy and applications of the following concepts:

1. That reading is translating a mark on paper into sound by a recognized system. That teaching a child thus to read is the *first* task of education and that instruction in comprehension is a *subsequent* one.

2. That the kindergarten program ought to make greater use of letter-like forms rather than pumpkin faces. That these forms should be identified and drawn. That coloring as now practiced has largely a recreational value.

3. That the first step in learning to read is to distinguish the shapes of letters. That the teacher should aid in this task by pointing out the difference between letters. That writing of letters, as well as seeing and hearing descriptions of them, is a useful tool in aiding discrimination. That emphasis be placed on the first and last letters of whole words that are learned.

4. That phonics—that is, training in letter-to-sound correspondences—should be introduced early in the instructional program rather than later. That this phonic program attack the irregularities of phonics from the outset. That the phonics be limited to the major elements of the language, with no notion of making the child into a linguistic expert.

5. That the child be instructed, actively rather than inductively, in the rules of spelling so that he becomes aware of spelling-to-sound correspondences that are the critical unit in the reading process.

6. That the look-say method has greatest value after spelling-to-sound correspondences are learned as a means of teaching pupils to recognize larger spelling-to-sound correspondences on an instantaneous or automatic basis.

7. That silent reading for meaning becomes most valuable at the point where reading becomes an automatic process, rather than in the early stages of reading.

8. That handwriting is a tool in reading instruction but of less value as a goal in itself.

Although we doubt it, we are willing to believe that these concepts may be in error. We are not willing to believe that they should not be investigated further and applied experimentally to classroom situations.

Regardless of whether this is done, we have presented this material to reveal some of the problems of the dyslexic child. We have seen in Chapter 5 the difficulty a child with perceptual limitations can have in recognizing the graphic symbols on a page. He will also have difficulties translating those symbols into sound. The reason for this is that the dyslexic child often has difficulties in recognizing and following sequential or repetitive patterns. For this child to learn spelling patterns or spelling-to-sound correspondences is often difficult. But as hard as it might be for him to be taught this, it is infinitely harder for him to figure it out inductively, as the normal child does. We believe that all children should be taught these spelling patterns and spelling-to-sound correspondences actively rather than inductively to speed the learning process. But to fail to do this for the dyslexic child with impaired visual perception is to guarantee positively that he will become a reading problem.

PART THREE

DYSLEXIA WITH VARIATIONS

7·

Research into Dyslexia and the Problem of Dominance

THERE AREN'T very many famous dyslexics in history. Obviously, a reading disorder is so debilitating that it becomes difficult to make a mark in a civilization that places such a high value on literacy. Macdonald Critchley commented on the comparative rarity with which adult dyslexics are diagnosed, saying, "Perhaps the patient and his parents have resigned themselves to a state of hopeless ineducability, and no longer importune doctors and teachers. Perhaps the victims have merged into the amorphous population of adult illiterates and semi-illiterates."[1]

There are a handful of prominent dyslexics, however. Prince Imperial, son of Napoleon III, was such a retarded reader that one suspects he was a dyslexic. A "reading machine" was constructed for him in a rather futile effort to help him with his lessons.

Perhaps the most celebrated individual suspected, at least, of having a neurological reading disorder was Hans Christian Andersen. For one reason or another he was a consistent failure in school as a boy. In his teens he earned a place with the Royal Theater in Denmark and his talents with puppets and his literary potential caught the eye of the king, who placed him under a royal tutor at age seventeen. Andersen was tutored for the next five years to the great discomfort of himself and the tutor. Most biographers indicate that Andersen could read, but his spelling left a great deal to be desired. His spelling errors were patiently corrected by his long-suffering publishers, but some of them remain, such as these from his diary following a visit to London in 1857:[2] Andersen spelled Shakespeare as both *Schakspeare* and

99

Schackspear; Macbeth as *Mackbeth* and *Machbeth.* Some others were *Manschester, Railrood, Saturdai, Roschester, brackfest, lungh, khatedral, Crismas, citty, rodindendron,* and *houscholds.* Gross spelling errors such as these are typical of a dysgraphia.

Knud Hermann, one of the leading authorities on dyslexia, has presented some accounts of the perils of dyslexia as reported by some of his adult Danish patients.[3] One described a childhood of school failure, pilfering and daydreaming, then wrote:

> Since I was good with children, I wished to be a teacher, but failed the entrance examination in Danish. I then obtained a post in a public office. In my spare time I had charge of a pack of Wolf Cubs, but when it came to signalling, the boys discovered my weakness and made fun of me, so that I gave up. In the office also they began to be sarcastic about my failing. I became heartily sick of their venomous remarks, resigned from my post and tried to be a domestic servant, but I was not cut out for that kind of work at all. Then I started at a training college for primary school teachers and worked like one possessed. I did well in all subjects except Danish. My essays were terrible, but my tutor then advised me to practice writing by copying. I copied a whole history of the world—that helped—and I ended by doing pretty well in my examination.

This patient reported to Hermann, "When I tell strangers that I am word-blind they will scarcely believe me. But I always carry a dictionary with me, and I never read anything aloud which I have not read previously."

Hermann also reported an account of an Englishwoman who was dyslexic.

> Perhaps I was twelve years of age when I started going daily to Queen's College in Harley Street. In the reading class there, each girl had to read out loud a paragraph of about two inches of rather small print. This lesson was simply agony to me. I dreaded it, my heart thumped from anxiety. I used to endeavor to sit in the back of the room and try to get the girl next to me to read my paragraph over to me in my ear, so that when my turn came I should know something about this wretched passage.

But this never worked too well, so the patient developed a better technique.

Just before my turn came I would scratch the inside of my nose and, having produced some blood, I was allowed to leave the room because "my nose was bleeding."

Another passage from this woman's account is interesting.

Not long after I married, in the course of conversation, my youngest brother said to my husband: "Oh, so you've discovered that she cannot read." I can read to myself very slowly. It is a physical effort. I tackle *The Times* daily. I think the shortness of the lines helps me, and I do not lose my place and my line quite so often as I do when reading a book. Constantly I have to read the lines several times to get the sense. I have to read each word by itself. . . . I am still very ashamed of my inability to read. I carry this dreadful secret always. I live in fear of having to read out something. At all costs I must conceal my ignorance—a habit which dates from my childhood.

She described turning down committee chairmanships because it would necessitate her reading aloud:

I realize I am now labeled a slacker, with no sense of duty, and selfish. . . . I am very fond of music and I belong to a choral society. We meet once a week and sing old and modern music. I am an alto, and I find reading the words and the music almost impossible—for I have not time and cannot keep up with the rest. I have to let the words go and learn them by heart at home. . . . My husband says cheerfully of me: "She's a very intelligent woman and a very badly educated one." My eldest brother says: "Considering how slow she was in reading and backward, it is wonderful how clever she is now. She always has originality and efficiency and does her jobs especially well." I have one child, born when I was forty years of age. . . . It has always been a grief to me not being able to read out loud to my girl, from her childhood upwards. I often tried.

In our practice, we have encountered several adult dyslexics. One was the father of a patient. He grew to manhood unable to read and found work as a common laborer—which was not overly challenging since his verbal IQ was measured at 135. He married a woman who could read and she taught him to recognize a few words such as *peas, beans* and *tomatoes.* This enabled him to improve his economic station in life by becoming a truck driver's helper. He would go through the warehouse until he found cartons labeled peas or beans and deliver them to the truck. He performed this work so well that his employer considered promoting him to dispatcher in the warehouse. But this was impossible, because he cannot read the names and addresses on the invoices. He remains one of the most intelligent truck driver's helpers in the land.

Recently a physician colleague, serving as a resident in pediatrics at one of the nation's leading hospitals, admitted in conversation that he was dyslexic. As he put it,

> I have an awful time reading. Always have had. I took every remedial-reading and speed-reading course known to man. None of them ever did any good. I wasted more time and effort trying to improve the impossible. I went through medical school and served my internship without finding the cause of my reading problem. Then a couple of weeks ago I learned about dyslexia. It certainly was a revelation to me.

When asked how slowly he read, the physician picked up a medical journal and said, "It'll take me about three hours to read one article in here. I'll work on this one journal during the evening for a whole week." That is slow reading. Normal readers would devour the whole journal in an evening or less. And a doctor, in order to keep abreast of his specialty, must read ten or twelve such medical journals a month. To be a physician, this man has had 12 years of public school, four years of college, four years of medical school, a year of internship and was on his second year of pediatric residency. During those years he has had to read hundreds of thousands, perhaps millions of words at an agonizingly slow rate.

What had prompted the conversation about dyslexia was a problem on which the resident sought advice. "I have a seventeen-year-old brother," he said, "and I know he has the same problem I have. I'd like to tell him so he won't waste all his time taking special reading courses. But I'm afraid if I tell him the truth, he'll give up and never go to college." It is hard to know what advice to give in such cases.

As this brief discussion of adult dyslexics shows, medical science has known about dyslexia for a long time. The first recorded mention of the loss of the ability to read was made by the

British physician, Lordat, in 1843, describing a transient loss he had experienced in 1825.* After that, many neurologists studied the location of functions in the brain. Hughlings Jackson and Broca are credited with localizing speech and other motor functions. In 1877, Kussmaul coined the term "word blindness," referring to the loss of the ability to read.

The first complete case study of dyslexia was reported in 1892 by the French neurologist, Joseph Déjerine. A patient of his lost the ability to read following a "stroke." The patient could write and record dictation, but could not read what he had written or any other written material. After the patient's death, Déjerine performed an autopsy, then reported the entire case, describing the brain lesion that had caused the reading loss.

In 1896 and 1897, the first descriptions of dyslexia in children were provided by Morgan and Kerr, who greatly influenced the writings of Hinshelwood in 1900 and 1917. These writers, as T. T. S. Ingram has observed,[5] were mostly ophthalmologists who paid more attention to visual imperception than to other clinical findings.

Hinshelwood described a family in which six cases of dyslexia occurred in two generations including four in one family of 11 children. In 1917 Hinshelwood described 31 cases of dyslexia and summarized the knowledge to that time. He defined "word blindness," as he called it, as "a congenital defect occurring in children with otherwise normal and undamaged brain, characterized by a disability in learning to read so great that it is manifestly due to a pathological condition and where the attempts to teach the child by ordinary methods have completely failed."

---

* Dr. Lordat described his reactions, as follows:[4] "Whilst retaining the memory of the significance of words heard, I had lost that of their visible signs. Syntax had disappeared along with words: the alphabet alone was left to me, but the function of the letter for the formation of words was a study yet to be made. When I wished to glance over the book which I was reading when my malady overcame me, I found it impossible to read the title. I shall not speak to you of my despair, you can imagine it. I had to spell out slowly most of the words, and I can tell you, by the way, how much I realized the absurdity of the spelling of our language. After several weeks of profound badness and resignation, I discovered whilst looking from a distance at the back of one of the volumes in my library that I was reading accurately the title *Hippocratis Opera*. This discovery caused me to shed tears of joy."

Hinshelwood observed that the disability occurred more commonly in boys than in girls and was often hereditary. The "blindness" might be confined to words or might involve words and letters. He felt the disorder resulted from the failure to develop the brain function concerned with visual memory of words, letters or figures. Auditory memory was commonly unaffected. Patients could usually copy written material because this did not require them to remember word and letter shapes, but they would be unable to write to dictation. Hinshelwood also noted the tendency of affected children to guess words they could not identify and to use pictures and other clues as to the contextual meaning. Finally, he felt the condition tended to improve as the children matured.

Several individuals made observations about dyslexic patients in the next few years, but the next large contribution was made by Orton, an American neurologist, in a paper in 1925 and a book in 1937. Orton made many observations of the way in which "word-blind" children, as they were still known, tended to make reversals of letters, confusing the *b* and *d*, and *p* and *q*. He also noted they reversed the order of letters in syllables and words or of syllables in words and sentences. Thus "the man saw a red dog" might be misread as "a red god was the man."

In writing, similar confusions were noted by Orton. Letters were often malformed and were frequently reversed wholly or in part. The order of syllables of words was reversed and spelling was inaccurate. He also felt that mirror reading and writing were more easily performed by dyslexic patients than unaffected ones.

Orton also described visual-field defects, that is, the inability to see to one side of a field of vision. He theorized that the dyslexic child had an inability to see in one-half of the visual field. This is now known to be incorrect. The mistake here was that Orton applied to children an observation which had been made in adults who had lost the ability to read as a result of "strokes" or other processes. As Orton put it, "The symptoms observed are a very exact counterpart of those seen in corresponding syndromes in the adult."[6]

Neurologist Macdonald Critchley has pointed out[7] the pitfalls in comparing a child who has a developmental dyslexia with an adult who acquired a dyslexia following illness or injury:

There are profound differences, psychological, linguistic and philosophical, between the problem of a developmental dyslexic, and that of an adult who has long ago acquired language in the usual way and then lost it. The latter has been using it as a communicative tool for so many years that he has developed his own individual associations and has unwittingly built up a veritable idiolect. His vocabulary—available as well as practical—is rich, extensive and replete with memory-traces. The linguistic armamentarium may even include patterns from other cultures, as well as certain non-verbal systems of communication. Language has thus grown to be an integral part of his personality, and his use of language has become a highly specific aspect of his total behavior. In such a person, circumscribed brain disease may impair this complex patterning, but the effect will bear only a superficial resemblance to the child who is slow in achieving this same faculty.

Dr. Critchley pointed out some of the specific differences, then continued:

> It is still necessary to emphasize these points despite the fact that they were clearly stated as long ago as 1903 at the Société de Neurologie de Paris, when R. Foerster presented the case of an imbecile who could not read. In the discussion which ensued, the topic was raised of illiteracy among children. Mme. [Augusta] Déjerine stressed that it was important not to confuse the pathological loss of a function with the cases of absence of that function.

The next major contributor was Halgren, from Sweden, who used the word "dyslexia."[8] He observed the genetic background of the dyslexic, making extensive studies of many cases. Since there is often a pronounced genetic tendency to dyslexia, his contribution was most valuable. Unfortunately, there are also many cases of dyslexia which are not genetic.

In 1950, Vernon's book on backwardness in reading was published.[9] The work by Vernon, a British psychologist, is important because she is one of the world's leading authorities on the psychological study of visual perception, but as can be seen by the foregoing, we do not agree with her central thesis that dyslexia is not produced by neurologic defect.

Chronologically, the next major contributor was A. L. Drew, who sought in 1956 to review the findings to seek the neurological origins of dyslexia.[10] He attempted to explain it "as a disturbance in Gestalt function which is inherited as a dominant trait. There is some reason to believe that delayed development of the parietal lobes is the anatomical substate of this disturbance in Gestalt recognition." In the same writing he said:

> If viewed as defects in Gestalt function many of the reported correlates of reading disability become comprehensible as parts of a single fundamental defect. Reversals, mirror-writing, mixed hand-eye preference, spatial disorientation, phonetic disintegration and other abnormalities often considered basic in congenital dyslexia are best viewed as variant manifestations of the fundamental defect in correct figure-ground recognition in both familial and non-familial congenital dyslexia. Attempts to comprehend and statistically analyze case material in terms of any single observed abnormality have not been successful. It is believed that the inconsistencies, confusion and apparently diametrically opposed findings reported in the literature and observed clinically can best be resolved by interpreting the findings in a configurational setting.

Knud Hermann published his book, *Reading Disability,* in 1959.[11] He focused attention on the neurological bases of reading disability. He was also interested in developing ways to teach the dyslexic child:

> In schools an attempt is made by means of varied teaching to ensure the maximum benefit, the children learning to read according to a combination of various methods (e.g., phonetic, spelling and word-picture methods). The exclusive use of the word-picture method, which occurred for a period in Danish schools, was virtually catastrophic for word-blind children.

The most recent major investigator has been Macdonald Critchley, writing in 1963.[12] He calls attention to the fact that no one knows the cause(s) of dyslexia. In some patients it is genetic and in others nongenetic. In some individuals the disability is permanent and in others transient or developmental. He sees dyslexia as a symptom appearing in several different combinations. Critchley was also one of the first to express empathy for the plight of the dyslexic child, referring to a youngster who was electrocuted because he could not read the word *Danger.*

There now seems to be a fast-rising tide of interest in dyslexic children. A conference on dyslexia was held at Johns Hopkins University in Baltimore in 1961. What may become the clarion call to help the dyslexic child was sounded in 1964 by Dr. Eric Denhoff, in his presidential address to the American Academy of Cerebral Palsy.[13]

> We must be ready to expand current habilitation facilities to meet the needs of these handicapped children. We must develop new programs to anticipate the types of problems that will emerge ten years hence. There are indications that motor disturbances and cerebral palsy are becoming milder and that learning and adjustment problems are becoming more apparent. Is this academy concerned enough about the changing nature of neurologic impairments?

The answer, coming from members of the Academy and neurologists in general, is yes. Many clinics and schools have been established to diagnose and attempt to educate the dyslexic youngster. A national committee on dyslexia has been formed, headed by psychiatrist Archie A. Silver of New York University and hospital administrator Robert R. Roberts of Redding, California.[14] There was even a Presidential Commission on Dyslexia. Educators are now interested in dyslexia, but there is an immense way to go.

DOMINANCE: CAUSE OR EFFECT

One of the roadblocks on the way to aiding the dyslexic is the question of dominance first posed by Orton in 1937. "The view here presented," wrote Orton, "is that many of the delays and defects in development of the language function may arise from a deviation in the process of establishing unilateral brain superiority."[15] This concept that dyslexia is related to problems of hemisphere dominance was a sensation among educators. Orton's ideas were widely circulated and many studies have been devoted to the problems of "dominance."

The fascination with "dominance" is not hard to understand. Much of neurology is quite technical. It is difficult to know a little bit of it. Studying reading disorders inevitably leads to consideration of speech, hearing, central language and motor disabilities. Unless one is willing to devote years (if not a life-time) to studies of brain function, he is apt to stumble into a neurological maze. A seeming exception to this is dominance. One does not have to be a neurologist to grasp that the brain is divided into two hemispheres and that the left hemisphere controls the functions of the right side of the body and that the right hemisphere controls the left-side functions. Nor does one have to be a neurologist to look at a left-handed child and see that he is different. Blaming dyslexia on left-handedness or some disorder of dominance is a convenient explanation.

Serious problems result when one attempts to do this. One may ask a child with which hand he chooses to eat, write and throw; with which foot he kicks a football; which ear he uses to listen to the telephone. These questions can go on to great length, for there are exhaustive ways to measure dominance. The difficulty is that no one agrees on what combination of handedness, eyedness, etc. comprises dominance.

The question becomes more involved. The location of the speech function in the brain becomes a key factor. Theoretically, speech is located in the dominant hemisphere.* If a right-handed, right-eyed, right-footed, etc., individual has a stroke in the left or dominant hemisphere of the brain, he will be para-lyzed on the right side of his body and lose the ability to talk (become aphasic). In actuality, the theory breaks down. Studies have shown that if 100 individuals who are right-handed, right-eyed, etc., have a left-hemisphere stroke, at least 98 of them are unable to talk as well. But perhaps two of the 100 are still able to speak, indicating speech was not located in the dominant hemi-sphere. Similar studies of individuals who are left-handed, left-eyed, etc., produce a different result. If 100 sinistral individuals have a right-hemispheric stroke, more than 50 percent can still talk (the figure depending upon which studies one reads).

This single fact (and there are others just as conflicting) plays havoc with all theories of dominance—or, more accurately, makes nearly any theory of dominance acceptable. There are as many

---

* Use of the words *dominance* and *dominant* is regrettable, for it connotes a brain process that is inaccurate. Dominance implies that one hemisphere tells the other what to do. This is not the case at all. True, a diseased hemisphere can interfere with the functions of the other, but it doesn't tell it the wrong thing to do.

theories as there are people to theorize, but not one of them satisfactorily explains why 98 percent of the right-handed people have speech located in the dominant hemisphere and less than half the left-handed people are so arranged.

Explanations for this phenomenon have been sought by using the Wada Test, in which a compound that temporarily inhibits the functions of brain cells is introduced into the circulation of one side of the brain. By observing the temporary loss of function, the investigator is able to determine which functions are located in which brain hemisphere. Widespread studies with the Wada Test have added to the confusion concerning dominance. The results suggest speech and handedness may be interrelated, but the tests also show some functions of the brain are not so related.

Another problem with dominance as a quick explanation for dyslexia, then, is the absence of agreement about what constitutes dominance. Are brainedness (meaning speech control is located in the dominant hemisphere), handedness, eyedness, footedness to constitute dominance? As we have seen, there are many exceptions that defy explanation. There are many individuals with disorders of dominance who read and write expertly. The welter of exceptions has led to the shooting down of every theory that has been raised. The resultant frustration has led some educators to dismiss as insignificant reading disorders the whole concept of dominance, as well as the idea there are any neurologically based reading disorders.

But dominance is important. The simple observation of the number of dyslexics who are left-handed or have mixed dominance dictates consideration of dominance in the reading problem. Just because the knowledge now available is inconclusive should not lead to a dismissal of dominance or neurological learning disorders.

The question of dominance may be wide-open for study, but some points can be made. We can dismiss the old wives' tale that switching from left- to right-handedness results in "epilepsy." This is most definitely untrue. All the enforced switching does is frustrate the child. Just immobilize your dominant hand for awhile and see how frustrated you become.

We can also discuss the causes of handedness. It may be said that a person has a dominant hand for one of two reasons: either the choice was genetically determined or his ability to use one hand is better than his ability to use the other. In the latter case, the child may have undergone minimal brain dysfunction* in infancy that negated his genetically determined handedness and caused a switch to the hand he was better able to use. To illustrate: a child may be genetically left-handed at birth, but for some reason the cells in his right hemisphere do not function properly. The genetic instruction cannot be carried out. The child begins using properly functioning cells in the opposite hemisphere, thereby becoming right-handed.

What sort of dysfunction could cause this? At this time it is possible only to theorize. The dysfunction can be permanent or quite minimal and transient, as is thought to be most often the case. This minimal brain dysfunction is thought to occur very early in infancy, certainly before two years of age. Minimal brain dysfunction is not a result of fever, a bump on the head or any other minimal trauma. It may occur unnoticed by physician or parents. Whatever the cause, the dysfunction often corrects itself, usually leaving no permanent neurological dysfunction.**

We believe that a permanent record of this infant switch in handedness is frequently found in the measurements of the nails of thumbs and of great toes. It has long been observed that these nails are measurably (frequently by eyesight alone) larger on the dominant side. On a right-handed individual the right thumbnail is expected to be larger than the left, for example. There are those who suggest the nail is larger because the dominant hand is larger from greater use. This is not a suitable explanation, for a

---

* Many writers speak of "minimal brain *damage*." It has, in fact, become popular to refer to "brain damage" or the "brain-damaged child." We vigorously object to use of the word *damage*. It is a nonspecific term meaning everything and thereby nothing. It provides no description whatsoever of the nature of the dysfunction and leads the layman to conjure up a mental image of a contused and lacerated brain. This might be accurate in cases of serious head injury—for example, such as occur in a head-on automobile collision—but certainly not in the disorders such as dyslexia. Furthermore, the term *damage* intimates permanence, which is often not the case. Finally, the term can be used inaccurately by anyone.

** One can theorize that the dysfunction might be a simple delay in maturation of certain cells. The tardiness might be sufficient to cause a switch in handedness. Another pertinent observation is that, while children normally make a choice of handedness by age three, some children do not make a choice until they are six or seven. Whether this delay is caused by a switch in handedness has not been determined.

significant percentage of individuals have larger thumbnails on their nondominant hand. If use alone dictated nail size, this would not be the case. Observations and measurements we have made of nail size of many dyslexic children show that roughly one-half of them have a discrepancy between nail size and handedness. The thumbnail on the dominant hand is either smaller or of equal size compared to the thumb nail on the nondominant hand. The same is true of the great toenail. Furthermore, these studies show a family history of discrepancy of handedness.*

The relationship between nail size and handedness is not an idle curiosity. During his years at the Montreal Neurologic Institute, Dr. Wilder Penfield localized an area of the brain which affects the change in growth of body extremities.[16] It is significant that this area is in the parietal lobe of the brain in proximity to other areas affecting motor, speech, reading and other abilities.

It is possible to hypothesize then that a large portion of dyslexic children had a problem, perhaps minimal brain dysfunction, on one side of the brain that caused a shift of handedness. The same problem that caused the shift of handedness also caused the problems in perception that resulted in dyslexia. Nearly all researchers admit such an event in the brain. We believe this to be the case in the less severe brain dysfunction, such as dyslexia. This theory of infantile brain dysfunction permits explanation of some of the perplexities which have been observed. Neurological disabilities could be transient or permanent in nature, genetic or acquired in origin, depending upon the form of the initial dysfunction. One, several or all of the observed phenomena, such as disordered dominance, unusual growth patterns, perceptual difficulties, speech disorders, impairments in motor ability, could be explained by the nature and extent of the original dysfunction. Children may have one, several or all of these disabilities. There seem to be infinite combinations of them. Since all of these functions are located in a relatively small area of the brain, it seems logical to conclude that an infantile dysfunction, frequently unobserved and of unknown origin, affected all, one or combinations of the functions to varying degrees and with varying permanence.

* Thumbsucking is not a factor in determining nail size.

It is our belief, then, that disordered dominance is not a cause of neurological reading disorders, but an effect of the same neurological process that caused the reading disability. It is a mistake, we believe, to view disordered dominance as a cause of dyslexia. Rather it is related, as another sign of the same basic neurological impairment.

Others share this view.[17] Lord Russell Brain, one of the world's leading neurologists, has written, "It is probable that in such cases the failure to establish a dominant hemisphere is the result and not the cause of congenital abnormalities of brain function which also express themselves in disabilities of speech, reading and writing."[18]

Psychologist O. L. Zangwill has written:[19]

> It is extremely difficult to understand why some ill-lateralized children have reading problems and others—almost certainly the great majority—do not. The first explanation that springs to mind is that both poorly developed laterality and reading backwardness where present together are due to the effects of an actual cerebral lesion. In cases with early damage to the left hemisphere, shift of hand-preference (either complete or partial) is not, of course, uncommon. Moreover, slow speech development and backwardness in reading are commonly found in such cases and may well be due to partial transfer of speech to the right hemisphere. . . . A second explanation is that a certain proportion of children with ill-defined laterality have in addition a constitutional weakness in maturation. . . . A third explanation is that individuals lacking strong and consistent lateral preferences (and perhaps also those with sinistral antecedents) are particularly vulnerable to the effects of *stress*. For instance, minimal brain injury at birth may affect more severely those who show no strong tendency to lateral specialization. . . . It is difficult to arrive at any very clear-cut conclusion. . . . The dyslexia itself may result from early brain injury, constitutional defect in maturation, or retardation secondary to stress. Indeed, it may well be due to a combination of these factors. At all events, fuller understanding of reading and its disorders must presuppose fuller understanding of the ways in which asymmetrical functions become established in the human brain.

As Zangwill suggests, the answers to the dominance question raised by Orton in 1937 are far from known. Much study remains to be done, but at this time we view disordered dominance as an effect of neurological disorders, not a cause.

We believe, too, that laterality of function should be observed in every examination for neurological learning disorders, and that nail size should be particularly noted. Nail size is the one mark left in the neurological sands. If a transient infantile dysfunction has occurred, all manifestations of it may have disappeared except the discrepancy in nail size. The child has switched handedness. His motor, speech and perceptual difficulties have cleared away. He is a normal child. Only the discrepancy in nail size remains as a telltale record of what has gone before.

Unfortunately, if the neurological effects of the dysfunction don't all clear away, particularly by age six when the child enters school, he may have some motor difficulty, resulting in poor coordination. His speech may be imprecise. And he may be dyslexic.

8.

Visual Imperception

THE INITIAL PROBLEM of the dyslexic child is that he is seldom recognized. Only when his reading disability is so severe that he is virtually incapacitated does he come before physicians and school psychologists, and even then the real cause of his disorder may be unrecognized. Most dyslexics are buried somewhere in the third reading group, where they remain on the wayside of education, an exasperation and source of guilt to their teachers, a disappointment to themselves and their parents.

In this and the chapters to follow we will try to provide parents and teachers with some clues which may lead them at least to suspect the various forms dyslexia takes. Parents can suspect, but it is the teacher who bears the primary responsibility for detecting the dyslexic child. She sees him day in and day out as he attempts to perform his school work. We are not suggesting that she diagnose his difficulty, only that she be alert enough to recognize a possible neurological cause for his reading problem and take steps to see that a correct diagnosis is made.

The next step is for this child to be tested by the school's reading clinic and/or psychologist. An analysis should be made of his visual perception and attention, his auditory perception and attention, and an evaluation should be made of his reading performance by various methods, including silent reading, recognizing vocabulary in isolation, understanding new words, oral reading of flashword recognition, speed of reading and comprehension. A history of his classroom difficulties in other subjects than in reading should be prepared, along with descriptions of his behavior and attitude.

The psychologist makes a vital contribution. He administers a battery of tests that provide information. Among the important ones are intelligence tests, which give a comparison of his intelligence with others of his age.* The psychologist hopefully uses the Bender-Gestalt test[1] for it is a primary means of measuring visual perception, as well as other tests. The psychologist also may make an evaluation of the child's emotional development. But the most important function of the psychologist is to provide an opinion on the nature of the child's reading disorder. He may recommend that a neurological examination be conducted. It is often wise at this point to have a pediatric examination and opinion on the child's general health.

When the child comes in for neurological examination, all of this psychological and educational evaluation, along with copies of his school papers, should accompany him. To say that this does not always occur is to make an understatement.

The first step in neurological examination is to obtain from the parents a history of birth and development of the child. This provides not only a measurement of the child's home life and possible emotional problems, but frequently indicates something of the nature of the neurological disorder. Obvious information to be learned is whether other members of the family have or have not had reading problems and disorders of dominance.

In diagnosing dyslexia we pay particular attention to his intelligence, for the first indication of a reading problem is awareness that a child reads at a level below that indicated by his intelligence.

The subject of intelligence automatically leads to the question of IQ testing. There is much popular and professional dissatisfaction with IQ tests. The New York City public-school system, among others, has discontinued the use of them. The disenchantment stems, in part, from observations such as these: a child has a high IQ and his teachers and parents expect great academic achievement from him. When he does poorly (or even as well as the average), his parents and teachers are disappointed and decide that IQ figures are untrustworthy. Or, a child has a low IQ and, the expectation of failure not withstanding, does well in school and belies the low-intelligence grouping in which he has

* We prefer the Wechsler test because it uses ten separate test units. This allows more accurate analysis of the child and his problem.

been placed. Observing this, parents and teachers decide that IQ tests are worthless. Or, the child of below-average IQ performs well in school, yet remains "sentenced" to a slow-learning group because of his IQ score.

These failings of IQ testing and the resultant criticisms stem from some unfortunate misconceptions. IQ tests are not measurements of basic intelligence. They are a means of comparing one child to others of his age group on a test which requires the use of intelligence. Dr. Kurt Glaser and Dr. Raymond L. Clemmens[2] have pointed out the dangers in measuring IQ scores in relation to a preconceived standard:

> A child with an IQ of 100, coming from an intellectually superior family, may be considered relatively retarded by his family and peers. Unrealistic academic expectations and pressures on the part of parents will conflict with the child's ability, leading to disappointment and defeatism. The school personnel may or may not reinforce the conflict by such statements as, "he is average—just like all the other children," and parents wishfully interpret this to mean "like his siblings and *some* children." Conversely, relative brightness may stand out if the child is born into an intellectually dull family. In such an environment he may not only suffer from under-stimulation, but may be actively discouraged in his intellectual endeavors which may be embarrassing and incomprehensible to his parents.

IQ is a comparison. Many factors may compensate for a lower IQ or negate a higher one, including ambition, motivation, physical health, emotional stress, family influence, cultural environment, etc.

A second misconception about IQ testing is the expectation of uniformity. IQ tests, like any other paramedical tests, are only as good as the person administering them. Suppose a psychologist administers a Wechsler or Stanford-Binet test° to a child who seems detached and inattentive. A good psychologist would expect the test scores to be lower than had the boy been more attentive and interested. Or, the youngster was very enthusiastic about the test. The psychologist would estimate that the score is probably higher than the child would achieve in an average situation.

° Wechsler Intelligence Scale for Children (WISC) and Stanford-Binet, Form L are the most common.

The problem with IQ testing is not the tests, but the use we make of them. It may be said that the tests are much better than we know how to use.* They are, most certainly, an invaluable tool in diagnosing reading disorders. We try, for example, to estimate IQ when examining a child. He is not labeled with a specific number, but an impression of his intelligence is formed from his conversation and conduct. This impression is then compared with his psychological testing. Suppose the test score is 75, which would place him in the educable-retarded range. On the score alone, he would be placed in special classes. But if the impression of the child is one of higher intelligence and that he might be fearful in a formal situation such as IQ testing, then a recommendation might be made to try to keep him in regular school classes rather than transfer him to a special education class.

The Wechsler test will also provide valuable indications as to the nature of his neurological disorder, for that test measures both Performance IQ and Verbal IQ. In a normal child these two scores are relatively close. But suppose a child has a verbal score which is ten or 12 points higher than his performance score. This leads to a suspicion of neurological difficulty. If his performance IQ is ten or 12 points higher than the verbal IQ, this suggests the child possibly has emotional problems or cultural deprivation. A low performance IQ may also indicate neurological motor deficiency, since the performance test is primarily a timed test involving motor ability. Clumsiness of the hand can affect the test score.**

The neurological examination includes (as indicated) the following: tests of muscle power, size and development; coordination and reflexes; observations and testing of handedness and footedness; tests of patterned motor activity; hearing, vision and speech; various forms of sensation. We often include reading, writing, spelling and arithmetic testing in the examination, as well as a few simple tests of various varieties of perception and other special functions.

Neurological examination of children with various learning

* This is not to say there is no room for improvement in the tests. It would be helpful if they were made useful in working with the culturally-deprived or foreign-speaking child.
** These are of necessity generalizations and as such are not totally accurate.

disorders seems deceptively simple. Most children enjoy it and consider it "playing games" with the doctor. It is usually a pleasurable experience for patient, parents and physician alike. Only uncommonly is there need for hospital or laboratory tests, such as electroencephalography. While useful in diagnosing some neurological disorders, such as seizures, analysis of brain waves rarely contributes to a diagnosis of reading disorders.

In this and succeeding chapters we will endeavor to show how the various forms of dyslexia may be recognized and how the diagnosis was made. The 32 case histories which are presented represent generally severe cases of dyslexia. The neurologist, at least at present, sees only the severe cases. Those which have been selected for presentation here are illustrative of the various forms of dyslexia. Milder cases, which would be much larger in number, would differ only in degree.

In our presentation, we have altered certain information to protect the identity of patients. Aside from this, these cases are reported in a clinical manner so that the significant facts which became known to us are presented to the reader. The most important of these facts include the child's sex, age, history, intelligence, school performance, handedness, and the results of those tests leading to a diagnosis of his dyslexia.

VISUAL IMPERCEPTION WITHOUT OTHER NEUROLOGICAL DEFECTS

The most common cause of neurological reading disability is impaired visual perception. The child has a brain dysfunction which inhibits his ability visually to appreciate and discriminate a shape and/or pattern. The visual-perceptual difficulty can occur as an isolated entity, or it can be seen in conjunction with one or more of the following: impaired tactile perception, faulty auditory perception, dysgraphia, dyscalculia, aphasia and other language disorders, poor coordination and other motor perform-ances, and the improper sense of direction and body image that are part of Gerstmann's Syndrome.

The disorder of visual perception may range from severe to minimal. The severe case is noticeable very early. He has difficulty discriminating letters from numbers throughout the first grade and cannot differentiate letters in the alphabet—something normal children are able to do before entering the first grade.

The mild case may not show up until the second or third grade. He appears to be just a slow reader who benefits from remedial reading. He knows all the letters in isolation, but when writing he tends to transpose their order in a word. He does well discriminating the first and last letters of a word, but the ones in the middle, particularly of longer words, pose more of a problem for him.

The child with mild visual-perceptual problems is more easily spotted on the basis of his spelling than reading. He tends to make "crazy" errors in spelling, making letter substitutions that aren't even close. The explanation for this is that in reading this child can "fudge." He "reads" by context, association, syntax, pictures and smudges on the page. He figures out logically what the word might be. In spelling he is on his own with little opportunity to "fudge"—unless he has had considerable phonic training.

The reason teachers and parents are wise to examine spelling papers carefully is that the child with impaired visual perception, whether severe or mild, has to retain a visual image of the word—unless he has had phonic training. He has to see the word in his mind, and visual memory for images is difficult for the child with poor visual perception.

Another way that teachers and parents can detect the mild case of visual-perceptual disability is to have the child read aloud. If the child is listened to carefully, it will be found that he gets the meaning and the context of the passage, but from time to time makes a word substitution that seems senseless. He doesn't know the word and he hasn't been able to figure out any clues, so he'll guess at it, arriving at *cheap* for *cheer, train* for *taught, mouse* for *music* and often much worse.

This fellow with mild problems in visual perception will learn to read, but he will be slow to learn and will always read slowly. He can often stay in the regular classroom, but he needs understanding of his problem and he needs help—help in discriminating and differentiating one letter from another, one word from another. More significantly, he needs phonics, as much of it as he can get. The look-say method is a disaster for him. He cannot spot the visual differences between letters and he cannot remember the image. He needs to make greater use of auditory perception through phonics and tactile perception through writing.

The alphabet poses difficulties for the child with visual-perceptual difficulties. He has special problems (and needs extra drill) on those letters which are rotations and reversals: *b* and *d*, *p* and *q*, *m* and *w*, *M* and *W*, *c* and *u*, *a* and *e*, *N* and *Z* (which is an N laid on its side), *S* and *Z*, *2* and *Z*, *1* and *I*. He tends to have trouble with *u* and *v*, *h* and *n*, *H* and *K*, *V* and *Y*. (This is by no means a complete list.)

This child has further difficulties in reversing the order of letters. He not uncommonly will reverse the whole word, particularly since English has a lot of words that make other words backwards, *god* for *dog*, *yam* for *may*, *tar* for *rat*, *deer* for *reed*, *dial* for *laid*. Not uncommonly, the child *appears* to read from right to left.

One of the reasons teachers and parents have had difficulty accepting that disorders of visual perception exist is the fact that normal children also make errors in reversals and rotations. There is a significant difference between the abnormal and the normal, however. The abnormal child makes more and worse errors, both quantitatively and qualitatively. The normal child is relatively easily trained out of his mistakes, while the abnormal child persists in making them long after others in the class have ceased to do so.

There are a number of ways of detecting a disorder of visual perception. Parts of the Wechsler IQ test, particularly the part using block designs, give an indication and the Kohs' Block test, which has the child make designs from blocks, may reveal perceptual problems.

The simplest and perhaps most useful test, though, is the Bender-Gestalt, wherein a child is asked to copy precisely and then, perhaps, to reproduce from memory standardized "geometric" forms. As in Illustration 13, there are nine designs, the reproduction of which requires perception of form, pattern and spatial relationships. A person's rendering of these figures can be graded by age. Thus, if a child of ten rendered these as a child of six normally would, a disorder of visual perception would certainly be indicated.

The following case histories are those of patients who have

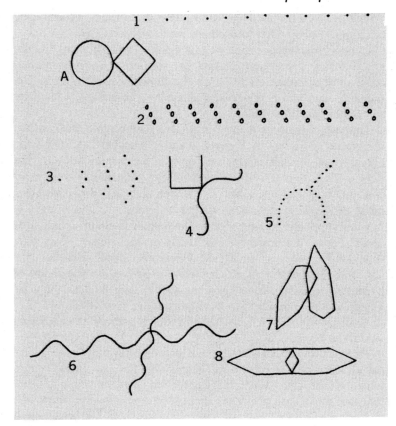

Illustration 13

impairment in visual perception without other neurological defects.

Case No. 1. F.B. A girl of seven referred by a physician because of her difficulty in school. She had, according to her mother, done poorly in kindergarten and had failed the first grade, despite an IQ of 112.

On examination one found her to be right-handed. The thumbnail of her right hand was larger than left, confirming neurological right-handedness. When tested for motor coordination and balance she did excellently. Her reaction to all the tests was to say, "I can't do that," before attempting to do them. After a little coaxing she proceeded to do them well.

Her hearing and eyesight were normal, as were both her tactile and auditory perception. In fact she seemed a perfectly normal child, until she was asked to copy the Bender-Gestalt figures. The depth of her problem is revealed in her renderings, which are reproduced in Illustration 14.

This was a truly amazing result. Her rendering of dots, which she made as dashes in Figures 1 and 3 was most striking. She also drew the small circles in Figure 2 as dashes, but saw the dots in Figure 5 as quite sizable circles. She had a very poor conception of Figures 4 and 6. Figures A, 7 and 8 revealed her great problem in detecting spatial relationship. The figures in A were supposed to just touch. She rendered them a half inch apart. Those of Figure 7 were nearly an inch apart when they should have overlapped. Figure 8 was also poorly drawn.

If this child had this much difficulty perceiving the shape of figures which are one to three inches in size, it could only be imagined the difficulty she had perceiving print in books. Endeavoring to teach her to identify the letters of the alphabet would not be very easy.

This girl was only seven and without other apparent neurological abnormality. It was to be hoped that her perception would improve with age. Meanwhile instruction in phonics and instruction that makes use of her tactile perception seemed in order. She was not a behavior problem, indicating that both her parents and teachers have been understanding and patient.

Case No. 2. S.W. was the youngest of seven children, all but the oldest two of whom had reading disorders. When seen, he had failed the first grade. He was a personable lad, bright and quick and willing to participate. A reading consultant who examined him gave an "All-American Boy" description, saying he was "a quiet, non-verbal boy during the testing, willing to do whatever was asked of him. He was somewhat restless with scratches and bites on his arm and face, and a runny nose. He cheered up considerably as time passed, then happily performed. Some of the non-academic measurements became games to him that he thoroughly enjoyed."

The reading consultant provided detailed descriptions of the

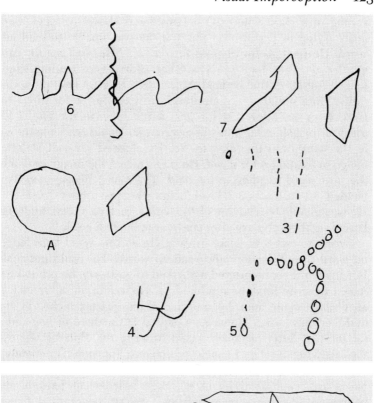

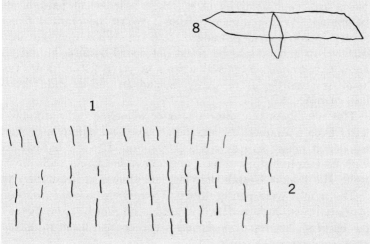

Illustration 14

testing of a child whose IQ is considered above average: "Seriously trying to perform on this test, he was unable to read any word. He read *go* for *dog*, *no* for *on*. . . . He read *tea* for *cart*, *you* for *dug*, *see* for *card*. His other efforts were reading single letters, initial, medial or final. More often he read final or medial rather than initial. . . . Samplings are *f* for *for*, *n* for *nip*, *l* for *Carl*, *s* for *as*, *t* for *it*, *t* for *left*, *k* for *Jack*, *w* for *saw*, *l* for *blind*, *a* for *ball*, *o* for *bone*. Sometimes he would read a letter not in the word, as *i* for *tar*, *i* for *to*. He showed reversal of letter image in reading *b* for *wend*. He then carried the image of *w* into the next word, reading *w* for *tend*. The Word Recognition Test yielded an instructional level below the pre-primer level. . . . He was unable to read any of the words, such as *a, ball, in, it*. He has no sight vocabulary after one year in the first grade."

Efforts to test S.W. were in vain. He had no word knowledge, no word discrimination, and read no words. He could not spell. For the word *go*, he printed *og*. Asked to write *my*, he printed *n2*. Asked to write *time*, he rendered *51*. His rendition of *street* was an oblong figure four by one and three-quarter inches in the middle of his paper. He wrote a capital *D* for the *b* of *boy* and *n* for the first letter of *make*. Asked to write the alphabet, he did the following: *a b c 3 2 f* (knew *g* came next but couldn't remember how to form it), *h i j K* (long pause, said couldn't write *l*), *m* (long pause and couldn't think of *n*), then twice went back to the beginning. Writing numerals from 1 to 10, he omitted 6 and reversed direction in forming *7, 8, 9, 10*. When numbers were dictated to him he said he could not do *26* because he did not know how to make 6; *25* was written as *51*; *31* as *41*; *31* dictated again was written as *13*; *42* as *24*; and he said he didn't know how to make *18*.

This intelligent boy after a year of schooling did not know a letter from a number. Examination showed no serious neurological deficit other than in visual perception. He was left-handed with no family history of left-handedness and larger nails on the right. His Bender-Gestalt drawings are shown in Illustration 15.

The figures were poorly drawn. There were marked disorders of spatial relationships. It will be observed that he drew figure 7 on top of 5, 4 on top of 3, started A and crossed it out to draw it another place on the paper.

This was a patient with a most serious disorder of visual

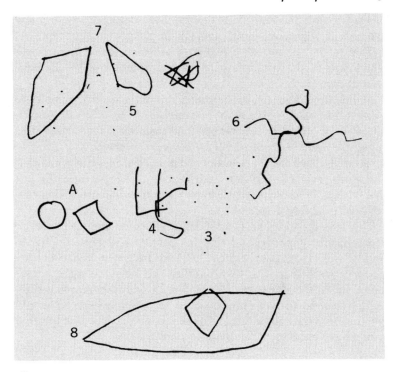

Illustration 15

perception, which is probably familial. There was hope for the future, in that his older siblings showed improvement as they grew older, some of them performing at grade level, as well as the absence of other associated neurologic disability.

Case No. 3. T.B., when seen, was ten and a half years old and in the fourth grade, having failed the first. He was the youngest of six children. The reading disorder may be genetic, as his mother was a poor reader.

He was a tall boy, slender, rather quiet and passive. On the Wechsler Intelligence Scale for Children his verbal IQ tested at 91 and his performance at 83, for a full scale of 86. The breakdown of the verbal tests showed he was in the slow-learner category in information, similarities, vocabulary and digit span, but average in comprehension and high average in arithmetic. In the performance tests he was in the educable-retarded range in picture completion and block design; slow learner in coding; low average in object assembly; average in picture arrangement.

This testing alone suggested a disorder in visual perception, which was further borne out in his reproduction of the Bender-Gestalt figures.

At this boy's age, it was supposed that he had shown improvement in his visual perception, but the degree of difficulty experienced in writing the alphabet from memory (Illustration 16) suggested that his future will be severely affected.

Observe that *l* and *k* are out of order; *r* resembles the *n;* the *u, t,* and *s* are reversed in order; and he was unable to form the last five letters. It is not hard to appreciate the difficulties this ten-year-old is having in school.

This was a child who needed help. He came from a family so economically impoverished that his parents had been unable to replace his eyeglasses which he had lost two years before. Chances were that with his disability and below-average intelligence he would never read well, but his visual-perceptual difficulties seemed to have improved to the point where he would respond to intensive tutoring. For economic reasons, this tutoring would have to be provided by the school system.

In these three cases we have tried to illustrate disorders of visual perception occurring without other neurological deficits and which seem to be genetic as well as non-genetic, permanent and (hopefully) transient.

For illustrative purposes, children with severe disorders were chosen, yet none of these cases is hopeless. Even assuming that no natural neurological maturation occurs, these youngsters can still be taught.

They need, first of all, time, a great deal more time than is permitted in the normal classroom, time for drill, time for trial and error, time to learn. They need a great deal of work on recognizing and differentiating the letters of the alphabet and simple words they form. They need to have their mistakes pointed out—patiently—again and again, and they need to have the unique characteristics of each letter pointed out to them repetitively.

Above all, as we have said, they need phonics, as much of it as they can get. The visual pathway into language comprehension

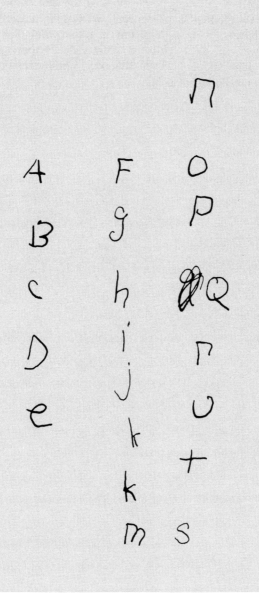

Illustration 16

does not function properly, therefore they need to make use of their excellent auditory perception. At the same time they need to learn through tactile perception, writing in a sandbox, feeling plastic letters, cutting them out in paper, and other kinesthetic techniques. In short, children with visual imperception can be taught, generally only with difficulty, but by regular classroom, look-say methods, not at all.

9.

Visual Imperception
with Tactile Imperception

IMPAIRED VISUAL PERCEPTION is frequently seen in conjunction with disordered tactile perception, that is, the child does not appreciate and discriminate the shape of an object which he touches.

Poor tactile perception, standing alone, is virtually never diagnosed, because it poses no problem in learning. It might make it difficult for a child to enter some occupations, but it will certainly not interfere with his learning to read and write and calculate. Similarly, when impaired tactile perception occurs with poor visual perception, it is not in itself debilitating. But we routinely test children for their tactile perception as a measurement of the extent of their neurological difficulties. It is also a clue to a possible means of teaching the child to read. All the youngsters in Chapter 8 could profit by tactile learning, by manipulating large cut-out letters and geometric shapes, fashioning letters with pipe cleaners, drawing in sandboxes and the other means pioneered by Grace Fernald. If the child has poor tactile perception as well as a visual imperception, these techniques will not be particularly helpful.

We test graphesthesia as suggested by the German neurologist Foerster, to measure tactile perception. The test is performed by writing simple digits on the patient's fingerpads while his eyes are closed. If he correctly identifies the figures that are drawn, he has no tactile imperception. The test is normally done on fingers of both hands, for some children have better perception on one hand than on the other. Sometimes it is necessary that the test be done by drawing a large number on the palm of the hand when correct identification cannot be made of numbers drawn on the fingerpad.

We routinely make a further test of stereognostic ability. In this, the child is handed an object while his eyes are closed and asked to identify it. He moves it around in his fingers and from its weight, shape and texture he is expected to identify it as, say, a paper clip. This is not so easy as it sounds. Stereognostic ability involves a highly integrated form of sensation. Poor stereognostic ability is uncommon, although impaired graphesthesia is seen more frequently.

Even less common, but most interesting, are those children with a *nominal aphasia*. When feeling the paper clip in his fingers, the child knows what it is and can state its use, but cannot *name* it.

This difficulty in naming an object led Knud Hermann to conclude that the child with poor visual perception perceived correctly but *incorrectly named* what he saw. As Hermann put it, "A *d* is perceived visually as *d* even though it becomes called *b;* the *d* is perceived as a figure with its loop on the left, but is named incorrectly. It is not, as some seem to think, a case of the letter in the process of perception in the brain being turned around and seen as its mirror image."[1]

We cannot agree with Hermann in this. There is no way to test his thesis with visual perception, but it can be tested with tactile perception. In testing graphesthesia, we often have the subject draw the figure which was traced on his fingerpad, rather than name it. There is no opportunity to label it incorrectly. It is amazing the reversals and "Gestalt equivalents" patients draw, that is, if a 6 is traced on the fingerpads, a patient may draw a 9; or if a 3 is traced he may render an 8; or if a 2 is traced, he draws a 6 (in cursive writing of a 2, this is a reversal). In some cases a child may make a double error. For example, a 9 is traced. He draws a *d* and calls it a 6.

Illustration 17 shows a rendering by a patient seven years of age, with very poor tactile perception. The bottom row of figures are the actual numbers that were drawn on her fingerpads, four on her right hand and three on her left. She was then asked to write, not orally identify, the numbers that were traced. The results, which are produced in the top row, indicate that her failure is not nominal, but actual. She got only the 3 on her right

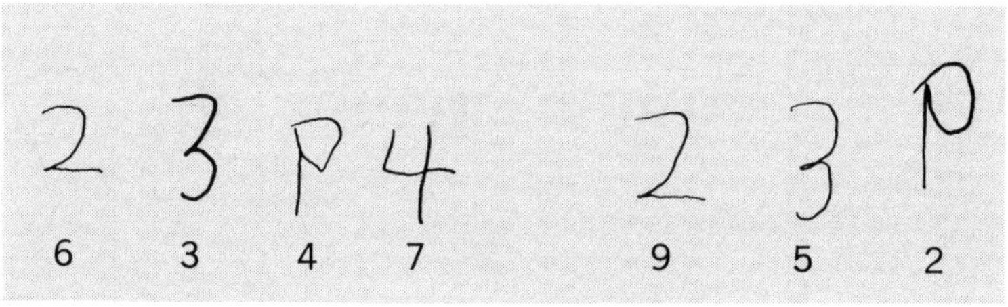

Illustration 17

hand correct. On her right hand she called a 6 a 2 and on her left hand the 2 was made into a reversed 9 or *p*. The 9 was written as a 2. The perseveration or repetition on the two sides is not understood.

Case No. 4. P.D. was a child seven and a half years old. He failed the first grade—allegedly because he was immature. In repeating the grade, he seemed more mature to his teacher, but was still unable to read satisfactorily. Reports from both his teacher and psychological testing showed that he had no visual memory for words. In contrast, his auditory memory was excellent. He used his above-average intelligence to read by context and by guessing. He listened to other children and the teacher read and quickly memorized an entire reader.

There were indications of a familial pattern in P.D.'s difficulty. None of his maternal relatives had any reading problems, but the patient's father reads quite poorly and haltingly. He reported leaving school in the seventh grade at age fifteen because of his difficulty in reading. As an adult he was able to read well enough to carry on normal activities, but he would often ask his wife to read newspaper articles to him.

P.D. had a great deal of neurological difficulty. His visual perception, as indicated in his Bender-Gestalt drawings in Illustration 18 was quite poor.

He also had some minor motor difficulties. His principal problem other than visual was a nearly total absence of tactile perception. He was unable to identify any numbers drawn on his fingerpads, although his stereognostic performance was satisfactory.

This patient was beginning to be most sensitive about his reading difficulty, a harbinger of eventual emotional difficulties.

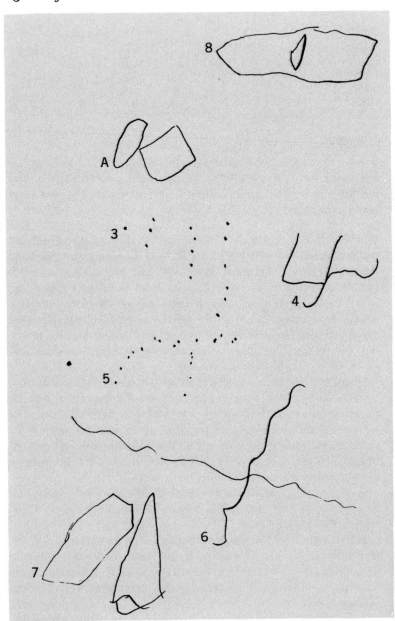

Illustration 18

His family, when they became aware of his need for private tutoring, particularly in phonics, arranged to have a relative who was a first-grade teacher give him private instruction.

Case No. 5. R.T. was a ten-and-a-half-year-old fourth-grader who not only had a great deal of neurological difficulty, but had been mishandled rather badly in school. In kindergarten his teacher observed that he needed insistent prodding to complete projects. His work habits in the first grade were also poor, and he appeared babyish to his teacher. At the end of the first grade he was reading at the pre-primer level—with difficulty—and had trouble recognizing numbers past ten. His handwriting was poor. Nonetheless, he was passed to the second grade. There his work habits improved, but he failed to pass because of his poor reading. This difficulty remained in the third grade and in the fourth, but his arithmetic was above average.

R.T.'s parents felt there was something wrong with him and so did his teachers. An effort was made to have him tested at the reading diagnostic center operated by his school system. He was on the list for two years before he was tested, at age eight. The center discovered he had an IQ of 112 on the Stanford-Binet. He was best in his abstract-reasoning ability and verbal comprehension. He was weak, however, in his visual memory for words and in hearing sounds in words, performing both at the mid-first-grade level. The examiner reported he had a "severe retardation in visual memory for symbolic material, greatly affected by lack of recognition of letter names and letter reversals." In reading the first pre-primer he read *apple* as *ball* and painfully recognized *got* and *can*. Later, when tested in the third pre-primer, he was unable to recognize *can*. In reading in the primer he made occasional repetitions and frequent omissions. He performed in a halting manner with much pointing to words as he tried to figure them out.

The reading clinicians did an excellent job of diagnosing R.T.'s reading problem—although they erred in recommending an emphasis on tactile learning, because they were unaware of his tactile difficulties. The clinic suggested that he be placed in a special reading program or have private tutoring. At considerable financial sacrifice, the parents employed a tutor, who asked that a neurological examination be conducted.

This patient's problems were probably genetic in origin. He had an older brother who repeated the sixth grade for a reading problem and a younger sister, one of twins, who had similar problems. The father reads poorly, having stopped school at age sixteen and thereafter attending vocational school. As an adult he had to ask his wife for the pronunciation and meaning of some words. He was told at a reading clinic that he was unable to learn to read by a sight method.

When seen, the patient had mixed hand use. He wrote and ate right-handed, but threw left-handed. The nails, however, on his right thumb and right great toe were larger and the family history was exclusively right-handed. He had no motor difficulties, but his visual perception was quite impaired. Halfway through his eleventh year of life he still confused *h* and *n*, *g* and *q*, *m* and *n* and several other combinations. Tactile perception was nonexistent on his left side and only slightly better on his right. His auditory perception was better than his visual and tactile, but was not normal.

Thus, this patient had an impairment of all three forms of perception used in reading. Fortunately, he had an excellent tutor, who understood the need to stress the phonic method. It seemed unlikely that he will ever be able to read normally.

Case No. 6. V.M. was a very rare child with a lot of neurological involvement. When seen, he was seven years old and repeating the first grade, where his teacher reported he had difficulty reading even the simplest words. His vocabulary was at the *four-year* level. There were very good reasons for this.

The first observation was that perhaps he had mixed handedness. He was right-handed, but his left thumbnail was larger. He had some minor motor difficulty. His visual perception was below normal, but not exaggeratedly poor for his age. This would not be an insurmountable problem were it not for the discoveries made when his tactile perception was tested. In testing graphesthesia, he was unable to identify a single digit drawn on his fingerpads or palms. Testing for stereognostic ability produced the following result:

A paper clip was placed in his hand when he had his eyes closed. He felt it and recognized it. "That's a . . . a-ah . . . oh-a . . . you know what I mean—a . . ." Asked again what it was, he tried again, "It's a . . . a thing . . . you know, one of those things you hook papers together with." Asked the specific name of it, he gave up, "I know, but I can't think of the name of it." Asked if it could be a paper clip, he said, "Yeah, that's it, a paper clip."

In another test, a small nail, about the size of a regular four-penny common nail, was placed in his hand. He felt it awhile, hesitated, then said, "It's a pen." Asked if he meant a fountain pen or a ballpoint pen, he replied, in some irritation, "No-no, a pen, a pen, the kind you hook cloth together with." Asked if he meant a "pin," he said, "I guess so."

At this point, the patient underwent a significant psychological change. The rapport which had been established disappeared and he felt defeated. To him it was the same old business about naming objects that his parents bothered him about. He was told to open his eyes and look at the object, and asked to identify it. "It's a pin," he said, "a big one." Asked if it could be a nail, he sighed, "I guess so."

This child had a nominal aphasia. His parents had observed this for a long time, but didn't know what it was or that it was significant. Instead he was rather thoroughly badgered when, sent to the kitchen for a fork, he'd return with a spoon. Sent again he'd come back with a knife. Three or four trips might be required before he brought the fork, apparently quite by accident. To send him to the store for a loaf of bread was, according to his mother, an invitation to the bizarre.

This was a most interesting patient. His disorders of visual and tactile perception alone would make it difficult for him to learn to read. Atop this he had the nominal aphasia, which meant he had trouble with his central language function, enough in itself to produce a neurological disorder of reading. It most certainly accounted for his very poor vocabulary which his teacher had observed. At his age, it was reasonable to hope his nominal aphasia was maturational and not permanent. But, consider how damaging to his psyche this whole process had been and will be.

Again we have presented severe cases, but all of these young-sters are teachable. As we have noted, tactile perception itself has little use in the customary reading process. There are only occasional subjects, such as art and industrial arts, where impaired tactile perception might be recognized.

The diagnosis is important, however, in preparing a suitable program of reading instruction. Endeavoring to teach the child kinesthetically is foolish. It can only intensify his sense of failure. The child who has impairments of both visual and tactile perception receives little benefit from writing as a learning method. He must be taught phonically, primarily. The greatest possible emphasis, the most patient drill must go into teaching the child the sounds of letters and words. Effort, of course, must be made to improve his ability to differentiate visually one letter from another, but the auditory process remains his best hope for learning to read.

10.

Visual Imperception with Dysgraphia

IN SIMPLEST TERMS, dysgraphia is disordered writing.[1] This should not be construed to mean untidy penmanship, for many dysgraphic individuals write quite legibly. The disordered writing of the dysgraphic is marked by faulty spelling and erratic formation of individual letters, as well as, sometimes, poor penmanship.

Writing disorders in children are difficult to discuss. They can conceivably occur in several ways and may be of more than one variety. Scholarly men, such as Macdonald Critchley, go into great detail, locating areas involved with writing in either the dominant or nondominant hemisphere of the brain. In adults great neurological significance is attached to handwriting. Neurologists look for lack of neatness, the spacing between letters and words, the size of the margins, and the slant of the handwriting as symptoms of various disorders of the central nervous system. For example, a person who writes only on the right half of a page, leaving a large margin on the left would be suspected of having a disorder in the nondominant parietal lobe.

But it is not easy to apply these same standards to children. Boys in particular are often quite untidy in writing, and every child has a certain amount of difficulty in forming letters. The ability improves with maturation, but the rates of development vary with each individual so that it is hard to decide when untidiness is maturational and when it is evidence of neurological impairment (or just the natural untidiness of a nine-year-old male).

If a child forms letters improperly, does that indicate he has dysgraphia or is it a product of poor visual perception? If he does not receive a correct visual image of what others have written, it is certain that he will not be cognizant of what he has written himself. He may not realize that he has put an extra loop in the *m* or reversed his *b* or rotated an *N*. Because of visual imperception, he may lack the image of a word that enables him to realize he has omitted or added letters.

There are infinite variations of dysgraphia among children who have dyslexia. A child with a mild dyslexia may deliberately misspell words to conceal his dyslexia, just as a normal person, uncertain of whether an *a* or an *e* is the proper letter in a word will form it inaccurately so it resembles both. There are all manner of variations in severity. A child may have a severe dyslexia and a mild dysgraphia or a mild dyslexia and a severe dysgraphia.

All of this is difficult to test. How much is dyslexia and how much is a true dysgraphia? Certainly, if his visual imperception is severe enough he will not be able to learn to write well enough ever to test whether he has any dysgraphia or not.

But, if dysgraphia poses a diagnostic problem for the neurologist, it is an asset for the teacher. Dyslexia, standing alone, is, as we have observed, somewhat easy for the child to conceal. He can "fudge," "fake," read from context, guess, slur words. A teacher can be fooled by the bright dyslexic. But dysgraphia is much harder to conceal. Writing itself is more difficult than reading, a double code with motor involvement. Too, in writing, the child must form a mental image of the letter and word. He is unable to use context as a guide. He is entirely on his own. Thus, the dyslexic is often more easily spotted by the teacher through his disordered writing.

The exposure which disordered writing brings to a child also makes this youngster more susceptible to emotional problems. He may be able to "fudge" his reading, but when he hands in his paper, he has revealed himself and his failings to the world. Writing is more traumatic for him than reading, and he goes to pieces quicker psychologically, as will be seen from the cases presented in this section.

In neurological examination, we try to obtain copies of the

child's school papers. These are usually illuminating. In addition, when we test tactile perception, we ask the child to write the numbers, and we have him sign his name to his Bender-Gestalt drawings. It is amazing the number of children with dysgraphia who misspell their own names.

Case No. 7. E.M. was a ten-year-old boy with a long history of school problems. When seen, he was attending an ungraded public school. The principal made the following comments: "He is working with a group of 22 pupils who are in their fourth, fifth or sixth years of schooling. This concept eliminates rigid grade lines and content designations. His class works in a Programmed Reading Program. It is a structured program and involves a phonetic approach to reading. Woven into this are the other facets of language—spelling, writing and English. Therefore, he does not have an independent spelling program. When I asked him recently to spell a word orally, he replied, 'I can't spell very well.'"

The principal reported that the patient had done well in his Programmed Reading Series, going from Book 2 in October to Book 15 in April. "His reading has improved, but he still uses an unorthodox position while reading and needs constant reassurance that he is doing well. He also has a tendency to reverse, insert and omit words."

An incident in class reported by his teacher gives some indication of emotional problems: "He refused to accept that an error was made by him on a multiple-choice answer even when he read from the story the correct verification of the answer. He insisted on applying his incorrect response to this excerpt. When shown the answer in the Teacher's Edition, he refused to accept that as valid and marked his paper as being correct. Four others had the correct answer and could not understand his behavior and persistence in arguing the matter because he had not acted so unreasonably in any other lesson."

Upon examination, the patient showed considerable evidence of discoordination and agitation. Both of these are on a neurological basis, but are probably transient. He seemed quite impulsive in his behavior, and his speech was not as good as one would expect for his age. His renderings of the Bender-Gestalt figures

(Illustration 19) were fair. His visual imperception is now quite minimal, which accounts for his rapid improvement in reading.

His dysgraphia was something else, however. In Illustration 20, he missed every answer on a reading test. His efforts are on the left and the corrections made by his teacher are on the right—including her own corrections of *apple*.

In Illustration 21, he again produced words which, while legible, are unintelligible. The teacher's explanation at the bottom of his work reads, "This was dictation of a paragraph and five sentences from his reading book. Although he can read this material and knows the letters which stand for sounds, he experiences great difficulty with written communication." Indeed he does.

This boy was best classified as a mild dyslexia with a severe dysgraphia.

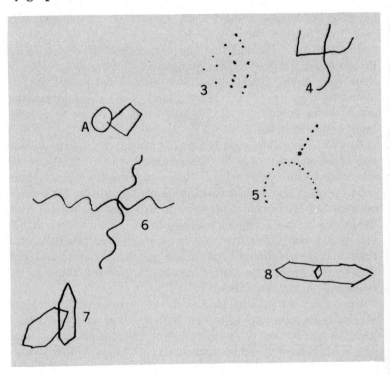

Illustration 19

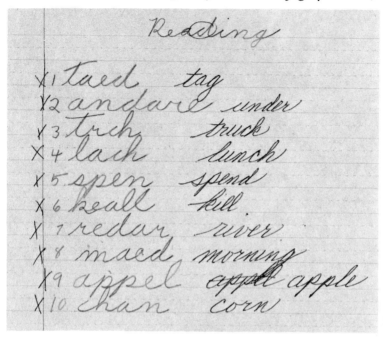

Illustration 20

Case No. 8. A.W. was a twelve-and-a-half-year-old girl attending a parochial school system. She had failed the second grade and, when seen, was in the process of failing the fifth grade. She had an IQ of 100 on the WISC, on which she was above average in testing for information, comprehension, vocabulary, coding and object assembly. Her visual imperception was indicated with an educable-retarded performance in block design and on her Bender-Gestalt renderings. These ranged from a nearly perfect rendering of some figures to an age-six performance on others. She appeared to have difficulty telling the difference between a dot and a circle. Her tactile perception was also poor.

The patient's dysgraphia is well illustrated in Illustrations 22, 23 and 24. In Illustration 22 it is difficult to decide what she was writing. The answer to question five appears to be "St. Gabriel, The Archangel" and in six it seems she was writing "The Ascension."

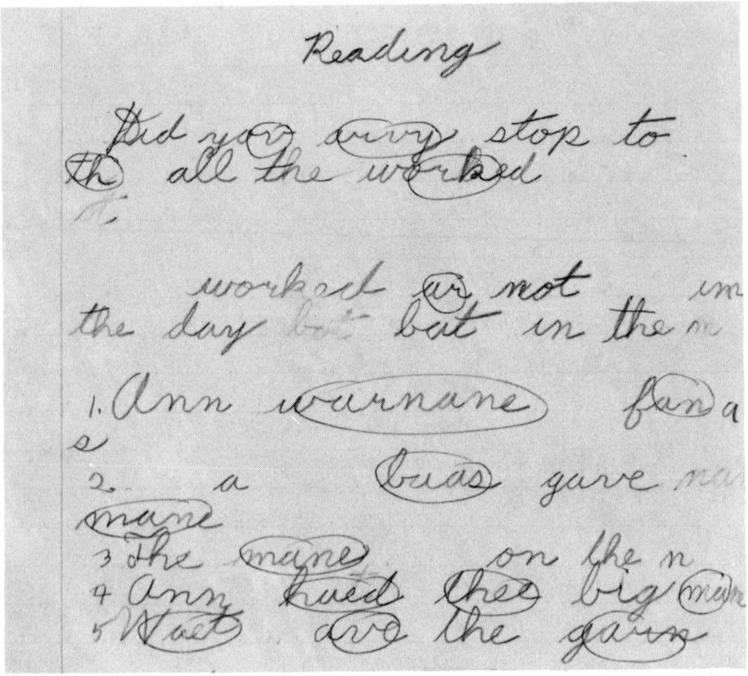

Illustration 21

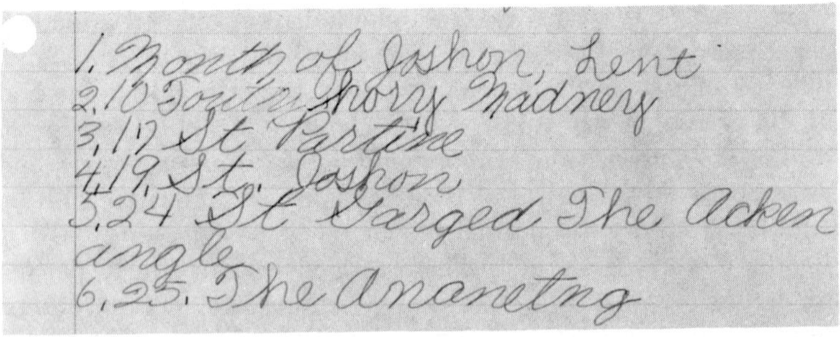

Illustration 22

In Illustration 23 she had some words correct, but most are unrecognizable. From question 19 on, it seems she was writing names of states, intending to write Kansas, Nebraska, Missouri, Minnesota, South Dakota, North Dakota and Montana, which came out *Ozerat*.

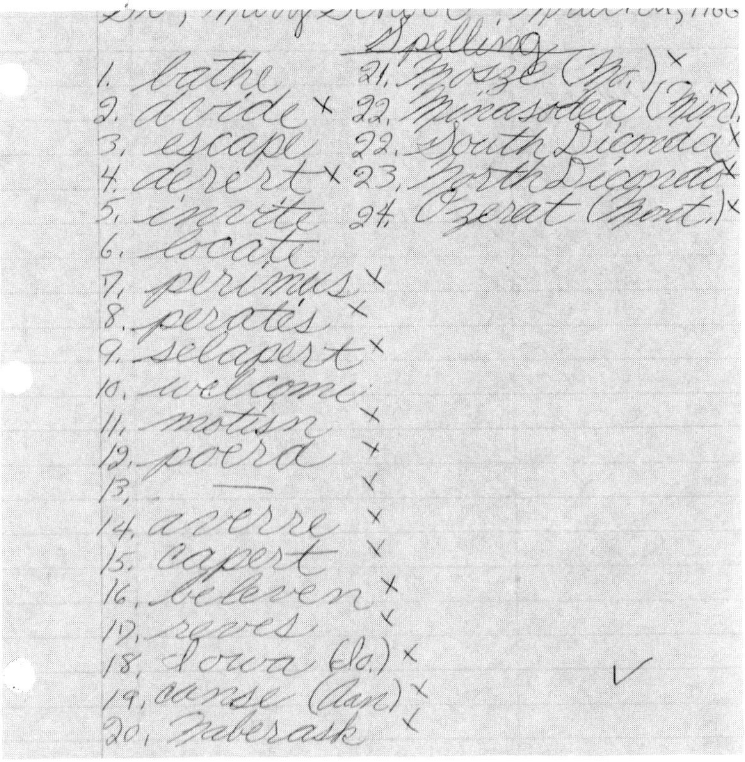

Illustration 23

These papers are good illustrations of dysgraphia. What the child has written is legible, but the spelling makes no sense. It is not even close, either visually or phonically. No teacher or parent should consider this child to be merely a poor speller.

This girl was a good example of how learning disorders can lead to emotional problems. She was of average intelligence, came from an economically secure home, and was quite pretty. But she sat in the office, her face wistful and sad, her hands clenched in her lap, peering incessantly at her knees. Her parents considered her quite a trial and were in great fear that she was mentally retarded. Her father was quite relieved to discover that she had good intelligence. It is significant that the mother did not accompany the child for examination, because she refused to accept the fact that her child had any difficulty at all and would

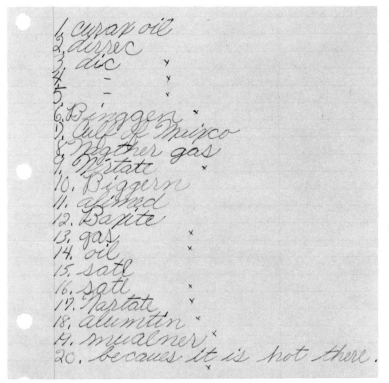

Illustration 24

make no effort to understand her. This mother's rejection was the child's greatest handicap.

Case No. 9. B.T. was an eleven-year-old fifth-grader who read at the second-grade level and spelled about as well. His IQ testing on WISC was rather illuminating. His verbal score was 82 and his performance 108 (26 points higher!) for a full scale of 94, just below average. He was rated as educable, mentally retarded in information, comprehension, arithmetic, similarities and vocabulary. His performance scores were average and above and he was superior in block design. All of this is a rather significant indication of neurological deficits in language and communication. His Bender-Gestalt testing was fair, indicating some deficiency in visual perception, but nothing serious. His tactile perception was all right and his motor ability was excellent. He possibly had some disorder in dominance, being right-handed while the nail on his left thumb was larger. His right toenail was larger, however.

Since no school papers were supplied, some testing for dysgraphia was performed. First he was asked to copy this sentence: "Listen to all corrections before transcribing." His efforts, first in printing and then cursive writing are shown in Illustration 25. He omitted a letter in printing *corrections*, but the effort was generally satisfactory.

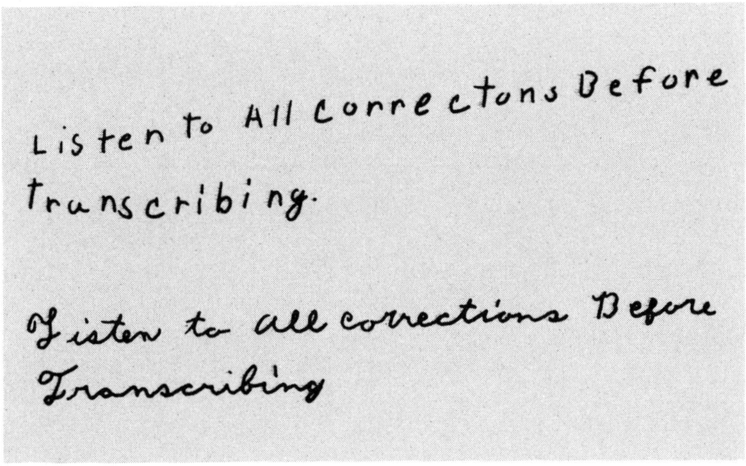

Illustration 25

Then he was asked to write the numbers from 1 to 10, then print and write the alphabet. His efforts (Illustration 26) were satisfactory for the numerals. In printing the alphabet he reversed the order of *M* and *N*. In his cursive version of the alphabet he made several errors; he reversed the *m* and *n*. When he looked at his efforts after he was finished he said the *u* (circled) "sounds like q" and said the *p* should be an *r*. The *o* is out of order and the *j* is upside down. It should be noticed that some letters are printed, both lower and upper case, and some are cursive.

Then the patient was asked to write three sentences describing what had occurred during the examination. His effort is shown in

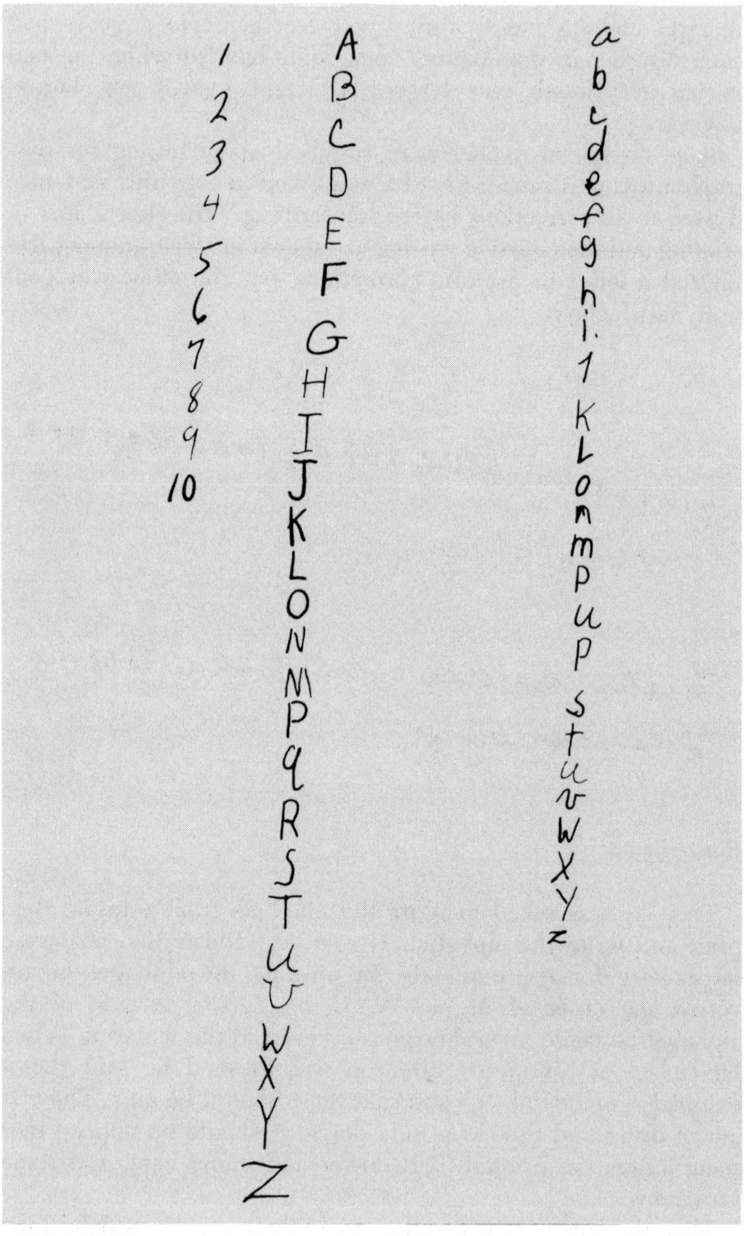

Illustration 26

Illustration 27. What, one might ask of this eleven-year-old, is *"manedert"* and *"nunedut"?* He was asked to read these sentences aloud. He said No. 1 was "we played games." No. 2 was, "He wrote numbers and I guessed the numbers." This was a reference to the testing of graphesthesia. No. 3, he said, was, "He put me in a room and I wrote sentences."

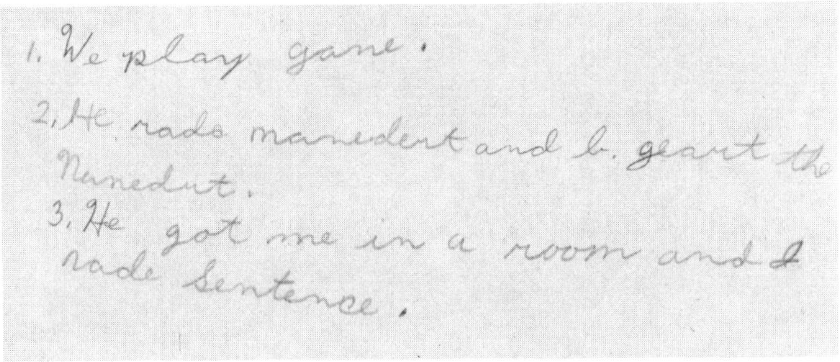

Illustration 27

This was a patient with a mild dyslexia, despite his grade-two reading level. His visual perception had undoubtedly improved, indicating that he could respond to intensive teaching. His biggest handicap was a severe dysgraphia when called upon to respond from memory. He copied satisfactorily. His memory for images when writing was so faulty that he had great difficulty with the alphabet. On less familiar material, he produced *manedert* and *nunedut* for the word *numbers*. On two separate occasions, he wrote the word *rade* for *wrote!*

This is an amazing case, an eleven-year-old child who can copy correctly, but who inconceivably butchers even simple English words when called upon to write from memory. One can easily imagine the puzzlement and consternation of his teachers! For a child of this age to have a problem of such severity indicates considerable permanence to the dysgraphia. He needs a great deal of help which can hardly be provided him in a regular fifth-grade classroom.

Case No. 10. T.C. was a twelve-year-old boy in the fifth grade of a parochial school, who produced a truly fantastic neurological performance. He demonstrated, in school, an obviously high intelligence which belied his record of poor performance—he was

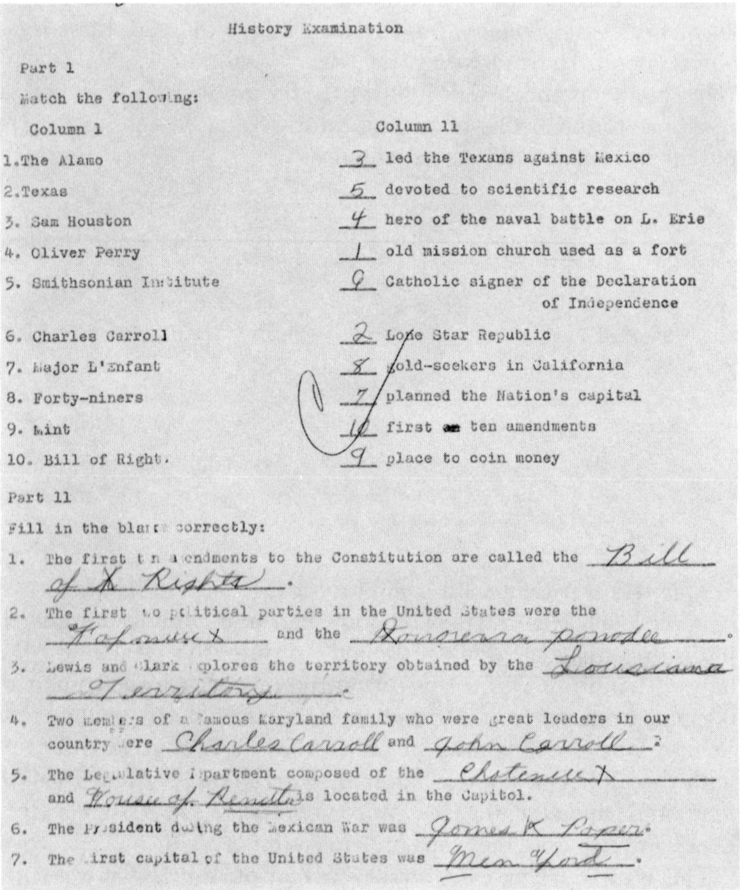

History Examination

Part 1

Match the following:

Column 1

1. The Alamo
2. Texas
3. Sam Houston
4. Oliver Perry
5. Smithsonian Institute
6. Charles Carroll
7. Major L'Enfant
8. Forty-niners
9. Mint
10. Bill of Rights

Column 11

_3_ led the Texans against Mexico
_5_ devoted to scientific research
_4_ hero of the naval battle on L. Erie
_1_ old mission church used as a fort
_6_ Catholic signer of the Declaration of Independence
_2_ Lone Star Republic
_8_ gold-seekers in California
_7_ planned the Nation's capital
_10_ first ten amendments
_9_ place to coin money

Part 11

Fill in the blanks correctly:

1. The first ten amendments to the Constitution are called the _Bill of the Rights_.
2. The first two political parties in the United States were the _Federalist_ and the _Democratic people_.
3. Lewis and Clark explored the territory obtained by the _Louisiana Territory_.
4. Two members of a famous Maryland family who were great leaders in our country were _Charles Carroll_ and _John Carroll_.
5. The Legislative department composed of the _Chotenusex_ and _House of Renst_ is located in the Capitol.
6. The President during the Mexican War was _James K Poser_.
7. The first capital of the United States was _New York_.

Illustration 28

failing the fifth grade for the second time. The Stanford-Binet test, administered in the third grade when he was nine, showed his IQ was 118. The psychologist who tested him reported: "His visual perception was excellent and memory for designs was excellent. He, based at the 9-year level, passed four out of six tests at the 10-year level, five out of six at the 11-year level and four out of six at the 12-year level. He scored 12 on the vocabulary which is one point higher than that required at the 10-year level."

With this great ability, why was he failing the fifth grade? Part of the difficulty was his reading. He was about a year behind, reading at the early fourth-grade level. Some years before, he had had a lisp, but this had cleared up, although when examined he was slow in talking. Some minor motor difficulties were indicated

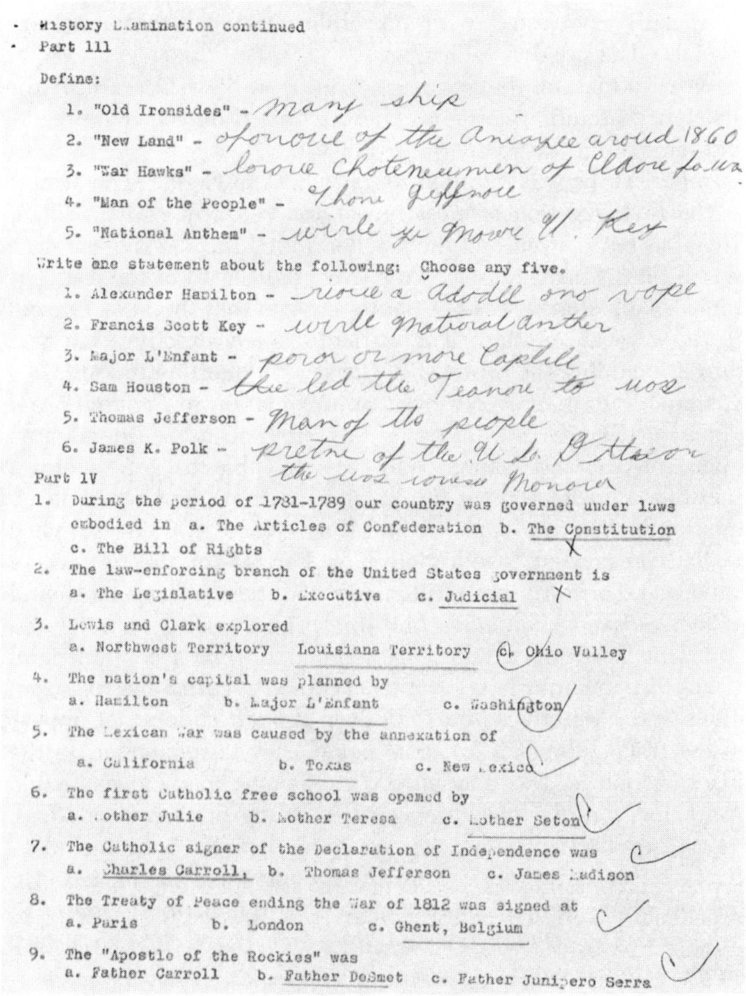

History Examination continued
Part 111

Define:
1. "Old Ironsides" - *many ship*
2. "New Land" - *of nouce of the aniogee aroud 1860*
3. "War Hawks" - *lorone Choteneumen of Eldoue fam*
4. "Man of the People" - *Thone Jeffnoue*
5. "National Anthem" - *wirle ze Mowre U. Key*

Write one statement about the following: Choose any five.
1. Alexander Hamilton - *niouce a adodel ono nope*
2. Francis Scott Key - *wirle matioual anther*
3. Major L'Enfant - *poror or more Caplill*
4. Sam Houston - *thu led ttle Teanoue to nos*
5. Thomas Jefferson - *Man of tts people*
6. James K. Polk - *pretne of the U S Ottaion the nos rouese Monoue*

Part 1V
1. During the period of 1781-1789 our country was governed under laws embodied in a. The Articles of Confederation b. The Constitution c. The Bill of Rights ✗
2. The law-enforcing branch of the United States government is a. The Legislative   b. Executive   c. Judicial ✗
3. Lewis and Clark explored a. Northwest Territory   Louisiana Territory   c. Ohio Valley
4. The nation's capital was planned by a. Hamilton   b. Major L'Enfant   c. Washington
5. The Mexican War was caused by the annexation of a. California   b. Texas   c. New Mexico
6. The first Catholic free school was opened by a. Mother Julie   b. Mother Teresa   c. Mother Seton
7. The Catholic signer of the Declaration of Independence was a. Charles Carroll,   b. Thomas Jefferson   c. James Madison
8. The Treaty of Peace ending the War of 1812 was signed at a. Paris   b. London   c. Ghent, Belgium
9. The "Apostle of the Rockies" was a. Father Carroll   b. Father DeSmet   c. Father Junipero Serra

Illustration 29

during examination, but his coordination was unusually good despite them.

This patient's neurological disorder was startlingly revealed in the test paper reproduced in Illustrations 28 and 29. Close examination of it revealed that this child could read, comprehend and copy accurately and was quite well informed about history. The test paper also revealed that he had a severe dysgraphia. It so sharply contrasted with his ability to read that it almost resembled a pure dysgraphia.

Observe that, on the first page of the test, he was correct in the first ten, matching questions. These required only that he read—and some of the words are quite difficult.

In Part II, he was required to *write* his knowledge. The answer to the first question is most revealing. The boy wrote *"Bill of Right"* as his answer, and the teacher added the *s* at the end. The reason for his mistake is shown in No. 10 of Part I of the test. The mimeograph stencil was cut improperly, so that the final *s* in *Bill of Rights* was omitted. The patient copied exactly what was above, including the mistake. In the second question in Part II he was unable to give even a close approximation to *Federalist* and *Democrat-Republican*. These words are not to be found anywhere on the test paper. Why was he able to get the third question correct? It may be observed that he first wrote in an apparently incorrect answer, and then erased it, doing so when he had progressed to question 3 on Part IV of the test where *Louisiana Territory* was written. He doubtlessly knew he should write *Louisiana Purchase*, but this bright young man figured *Louisiana Territory* would be close enough to be acceptable, and it was. In the fourth question he copied *Charles Carroll* from above and correctly wrote *John* even though it does not appear on the test paper. It is a simple name, easy to remember. In the fifth question he was unable to write *Senate*, made a reasonable approximation of *House* but was hamstrung on *Representatives*.

On the sixth question, he missed *James K. Polk*—including the fact it was reproduced on the second page of the test. He knew it was a simple name though, and did his best—*Jomes K. Poper*. On the seventh question, he came fairly close to a very simple, familiar word.

On Part IV of the test he demonstrated that he is reasonably well-informed about history, but in Part III, his disability was revealed to all the world. He could write a few simple words, but most are unintelligible. Almost pathetic is his effort to produce *Thomas Jefferson.* He could have copied it, but it would appear that by this time he was so desperate and disturbed by his obvious failure—he can read and thus knows he is not writing words correctly—that the system which had worked for him at the outset of the test had broken down.

During his neurological examination, we asked him to write some words. In Illustration 30, his efforts to write *Mexico, Congress* and *Senate* are reproduced:

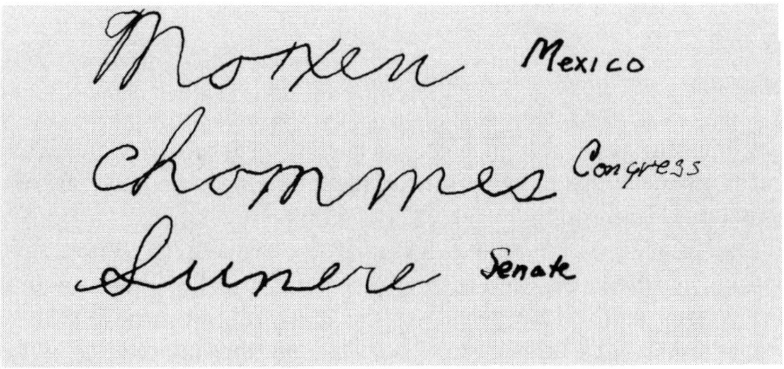

Illustration 30

Then, he was asked to copy the names of four states. We wrote the states and he copied them. In Illustration 31, it may be seen that he did quite well, erring only in the *n* in *Maryland.*

Then the paper was folded and he was asked to write from memory the four states which he had just written. His effort (Illustration 32) shows how fleeting his visual memory was. *Texas* and *Virginia* are barely recognizable. *Maryland,* his home state, is only slightly wrong, and *Ohio,* a short, easily remembered word, is correct.

This patient has a serious dysgraphia. His performance at age twelve indicates a high degree of permanence to his disability. To continue to test this child by having him write and to grade this child on these tests and to measure his knowledge and scholastic ability by such tests are grossly unfair. The boy knows the answer, but he cannot write it—and never will. Nor is it neces-

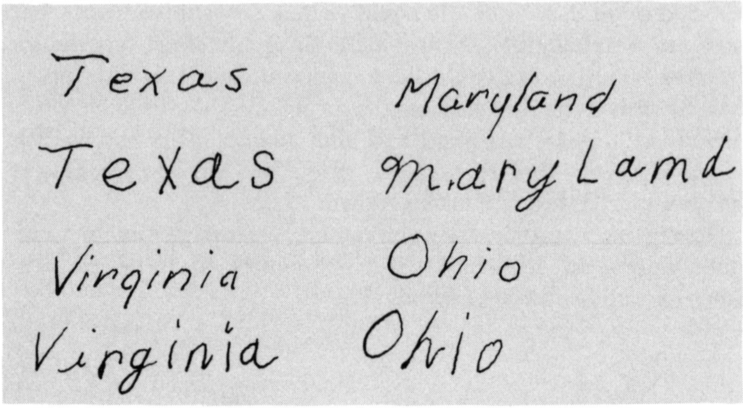

Illustration 31

sary for him to be able to write. A person with an IQ of 118 who can read can enter most technical and mercantile professions. All he needs is a secretary.

The educational demand for written answers to which this patient had been exposed during five years of school had exacted a psychological toll. He was largely defeated, not only in school but at home. His home was a broken one and his mother, with whom he lived, was impoverished and existing on charity. The psychologist who examined him said: "He is a sensitive child, a shy, insecure, very fine person. He is appreciative of what is done for him. He is embarrassed because his mother has to receive help. He is so embarrassed when food or clothing is brought to the home, he wants to run away. He is a likeable boy, to be pitied."

It must not be forgotten that the principal difficulty of some of

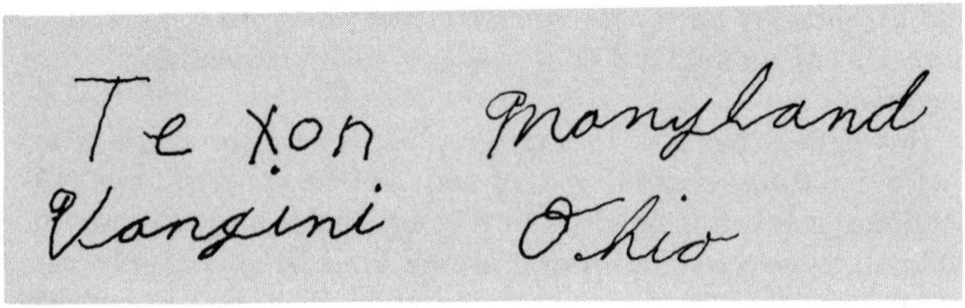

Illustration 32

the children described in this chapter is that they have faulty visual perception. This keeps them from recognizing their own spelling errors.

Correcting the visual imperception must be done in the manner we have already described, through drill in discriminating one letter from another, through intensive use of phonics, and through kinesthetic methods, if the child has no tactile imperception.

As for the dysgraphia, it is difficult to correct except as visual perception improves. Simple humanity dictates that less emphasis on writing be made with the dysgraphic child. As we have noted, he needs to be tested orally, instead of in writing. In some cases, simply teaching him to operate a typewriter can ease his difficulties.

Visual Imperception
with Gerstmann's Syndrome

ONE OF THE NOTEWORTHY EFFORTS to "explain" neurological reading disorders is Knud Hermann's theory that all are a juvenile manifestation of a congenital Gerstmann's syndrome.* Hermann wrote: "The many points of similarity between the symptoms of Gerstmann's syndrome and of constitutional dyslexia make it highly probable that congenital word-blindness is dependent on the same disturbance of directional function which is responsible for the symptoms of Gerstmann's syndrome."[1]

In the 1920's Josef Gerstmann described a syndrome in adults consisting of: (1) dysgraphia, (2) dyscalculia (disability in understanding or using numbers in arithmetic), (3) finger agnosia (disability in differentiating one's own fingers either by name or touch), and (4) right-left disorientation. This work has caused great excitement and discussion among neurologists and neuropsychologists ever since.**

Gerstmann made his observation in adults, and it was a significant contribution. There are such people, some of them acutely disabled. Hermann, because he observed similar symp-

---

* Syndrome: a group of signs and/or symptoms occurring together but not a disease and not resulting from one specific known origin.

** The finger agnosia may apply to other portions of the body in rare instances, but the more localized form is considered to be the more common. Whether right-left disorientation should be extended to include disordered "directional sense" is questionable. Lange, Stengel and Juba have applied Gestalt psychological theory to this directional disorder. It is in this way that Hermann[2] comes to regard the disturbance of directional function as the basic process in all four portions of Gerstmann's syndrome. Neither Gerstmann nor Critchley can agree.[3] Nor can we.

toms in children, theorized that all dyslexic children have a congenital Gerstmann's syndrome. In our view, as well as in the opinion of Critchley and others, Hermann added 2 and 2 and arrived at 22. There are children who have a reading disorder and several of the symptoms of Gerstmann's syndrome, and they will be the subject of this chapter. There are many other children—in fact, most other patients—who have a reading disorder and only one of the Gerstmann symptoms. They may have dyslexia and dysgraphia, but no disorders of calculation, direction, or body image. They may have a dyslexia and *no* other neurological disorders at all. Thus, the central phenomenon of neurological reading disorders—their great variety—remains.

In neurological examination, we regularly look for these symptoms of Gerstmann's syndrome. The dysgraphia and dyscalculia are rather easily diagnosed by having the child write and by examining his school papers. Dysgraphia has been described, but some explanation should be made of dyscalculia.

Standing alone as a disorder, dyscalculia is so seldom seen by neurologists that it is believed the disorder is rare. We are not certain this is the case. Gross difficulty in adding, subtracting, multiplying, dividing and in performing the higher forms of mathematics can be neurological in origin, as well as caused by poor teaching techniques, lack of pupil interest and below-average intelligence. It is certain that many students are less than brilliant in arithmetic, for one reason or another.

We suspect that a pure dyscalculia could be diagnosed by the nature of the child's mistakes. He would fail to grasp the principle behind the calculation. He would not be close in his answers, and he obviously would be guessing. The whole character of his calculation would differ from the child who was simply inexpert in his number facts.

We have never seen a pure dyscalculia.* It may be rare, but we suspect the child who is poor in arithmetic is simply less of an educational problem. He fails that subject, but if he reads and

* It can be conjectured that "dyscalculics" may start to appear in greater numbers as a result of the so-called new math, which deemphasizes rote memorization in favor of learning concepts involved in calculation. Only time will tell, but it may be expected that the new approach will pose more difficulty for the neurologically impaired child than simple memorization of number facts.

does well in other courses, he passes to the next grade and is viewed as a success in school. No one considers a neurological examination warranted.

Testing for finger agnosia can be most complex in adults. Neurologists sometimes go through involved procedures to determine the nature and extent of the disability. In children we do a rather simple procedure. We ask the patient to sit on a chair and put his hands on his thighs, palms down. If he cannot tell his left hand from his right, we will mark one with a strip of adhesive tape. Then he is instructed that the fingers of each hand are numbered, with the thumbs being 1 and the small finger 5. Now the patient closes his eyes. When one of his fingers is touched, the child is asked to identify it. For example the ring finger would be left 4. The middle finger on the right hand would be right 3. His fingers may be touched singly or in combinations.

As simple as this test is, the child with disordered body image will have difficulty performing it. He often confuses 3 and 4 when touched individually, or 2, 3 or 4 when touched simultaneously. For example, if 2 on one hand is touched and 4 on the other, he will frequently say that both 2's were touched. The patient also often confuses 1 and 5. If, for example, both thumbs were touched, he'll suggest that 1 and 5 were touched or perhaps that both were 5's. This type of performance is indicative of finger agnosia.

Disordered sense of right-left discrimination is often detected by such a simple procedure as asking a child which hand he writes with. He says his right hand but holds up his left. Or the child may be asked to touch his right eye with his left hand, or to touch the examiner's left eye, or, quickly to stand up and turn around to his left, sit down and wiggle his right foot and point to the examiner's right hand. There are many variations of these simple exercises, but whichever are used, they accomplish three purposes: the patient is asked (1) to point to a part of his body as directed; (2) to perform a movement that involves direction; and (3) to detect correctly a mirror image by pointing to an examiner's hand or eye. The test will vary with the age of the patient. A child in the second or third grade should be aware of direction in mirror images.

Right-left disorientation and finger agnosia can be inconveniencing and, if severe, disabling, but they seldom affect school performance. Poor direction sense may cause a child to read from right to left, perhaps, but, in general, teachers and parents would take little notice of the whole disability. But the symptoms of Gerstmann's syndrome are of interest to neurologists because they indicate the extent of the patient's neurological involvement. In children, however, one seldom sees Gerstmann's syndrome occurring as totally as in adults. Only one or two of the symptoms may be detected, but for want of better nomenclature we are saying that the patients in the following cases have symptoms of Gerstmann's syndrome along with impaired visual perception.

Case No. 11. C.N. was an eight-year, eight-month-old boy in the second grade who had a severe reading problem. He had considerable trouble learning the alphabet in the first grade and repeated it. In the second grade he still had a problem differentiating 6 and 9 when they were printed. The lower-case printing of *b* and *d*, *h* and *r* and other combinations bothered him. This was borne out when he substituted an *m* for an *n* in writing his last name. A reading examination administered to him at a clinic showed that more than halfway through his third year of schooling, he read orally at the mid-first-grade level, had a low sight vocabulary and made errors on such words as *a, the, it* and *to*. In testing for silent reading, he read at the first-grade level with no comprehension and with inaccurate recall and guesses.

This patient had neurologic abnormalities. He had a marked disorder in handedness. The nail on his left thumb was a full millimeter wider than his right thumbnail, yet he was right-handed. When he was in kindergarten, his medical records show, he sustained a bad laceration of his right wrist, severing the radial artery, all of the nerves in the wrist and many of the tendons to the hand. This was repaired surgically and amazingly satisfactorily, but during a whole year of healing, the patient used his left hand. When the right hand recovered its function and was no longer immobilized, he switched back to using his right hand. This is especially interesting since his tactile perception was markedly poorer on his right hand than his left.* We had the impression that he was genetically left-handed, but had a dysfunction in the right cerebral hemisphere that necessitated a

---

* Not due to the severed, now repaired, nerves.

switch to the right hand, where his performance was generally inferior.

He was able to perform satisfactorily all the various tests of motor coordination, but his ability to discriminate between left and right was inaccurate and slow. His ability to identify his fingers was poor and broke down completely when more than one finger was touched. And, he apparently had dyscalculia. His teacher reported he did poorly in arithmetic, not only failing to recognize the numbers, but also to grasp the arithmetical principle involved. Thus, this patient had all the symptoms of Gerstmann's syndrome.

Atop all of this he had mildly impaired visual perception, as witnessed by his Bender-Gestalt (Illustration 33). Not only are the figures poorly drawn, but they are all bunched on the left side of the page.*

The sheer weight of this child's neurological abnormality (and it should be pointed out that there was no familial history of similar disorders) made his a serious case—particularly since his nightly enuresis was evidence he was being affected psychologically.

Maintaining such a child in a normal class setting was to give up on him. He needed schooling with a special, daily emphasis on reading therapy, even then not a great deal could be done with him immediately. His future hinged on a slow and prolonged educational process requiring great patience.

Case No. 12. J.A. was a ten-and-one-half-year-old who repeated the first grade and was taking his second "crack" at the third grade, principally because he still read at the first-grade level. One needed to look no farther for a cause for this than his visual perception, which was most minimal, as indicated by his Bender-Gestalt renderings in Illustration 34.

For a boy halfway through his eleventh year of life, these renderings were quite bad and his reading was, too.

Neurological examination gave indication of other serious problems. He was right-handed, but the nail on his left thumb was larger. He had some motor difficulty, particularly when called upon to make both of his hands work together. It was not

---

* Critchley suggests that this is significant of disorder in the nondominant parietal cortex.

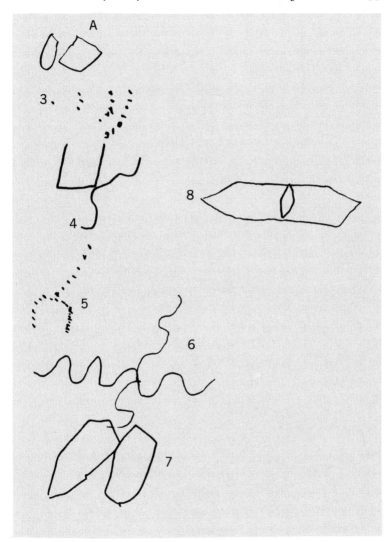

Illustration 33

surprising that his parents reported that it was only a year previously, at age 9½, that he had learned to tie his shoelaces and button his clothes. He showed considerable disorder in discriminating left from right, and he had mild finger agnosia.

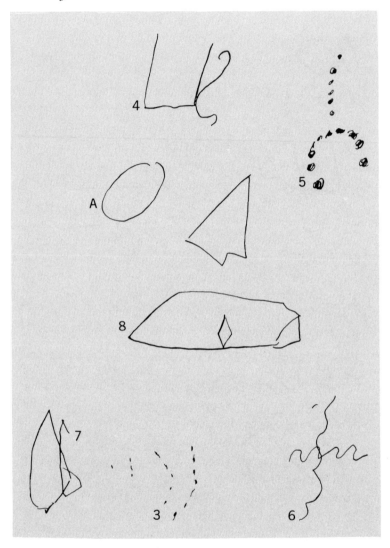

Illustration 34

For a child of this age to have all of this malfunction was regrettable. He would need as much individual reading instruction as possible for the next five to six years. But he could be taught to read, at least better than the first-grade level. It should be remembered that his reading disorder was primarily one of visual imperception. His symptoms of Gerstmann's syndrome and his motor difficulties, while they indicated a considerable neurological involvement and posed other problems in life for him, probably did not directly interfere with his learning to read.

Case No. 13. J.K. was a ten-and-a-half-year-old boy who repeated the first grade and, when seen, was in the third. His school teacher described him as "extremely poor in reading" and felt "he never worked to capacity," which, neurologically, was a matter open to dispute.

This patient was a good example of the difficulties school officials can have diagnosing a reading problem, unless some neurological information is obtained. He came from a good home, and he was in no way a behavior problem. His teacher described him as "well-accepted by the other children. He is anxious to please, desirous of improvement. He appears to like school." His IQ on the WISC was below average, with his verbal IQ at 90 and his performance a surprising 78. In the performance test he was in the educable-retarded range in block design and in the trainable-retarded in object assembly. In the verbal tests he was quite poor in detecting similarities, but well above average in comprehension.

The root of his reading problem was perceptual, which showed in his Bender-Gestalt drawings in Illustration 35.

He had more wrong with him than poor visual perception, however. He had a severe finger agnosia and some left-right confusion. On top of that he had a great problem with tactile perception, particularly on the right side—and he was right-handed. His motor coordination was also poor, particularly when he was asked to do different tasks with each hand at the same time.

This patient's school history indicated that his difficulty was not so much that he was not working up to his capacity, but that the school was not making use of what capacities he had. During his first two years, he was taught in a school which used an almost pure look-say method of reading instruction. He was constantly admonished to recognize the pattern that a word makes. With his impaired visual perception and his problems in motor pattern, this was a most difficult task for him. He was

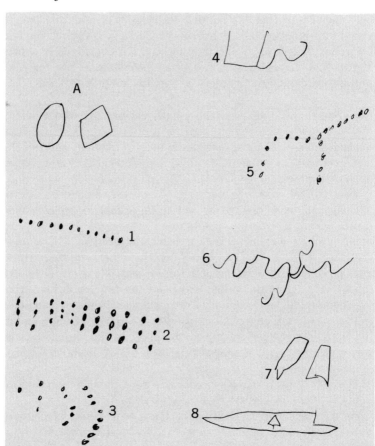

Illustration 35

taught virtually no phonics, and it was precisely this that he quite desperately needed if he was ever going to read.

Case No. 14. C.Y. was a nine-and-a-half-year-old girl in the third grade who had repeated the second. Interestingly, she was not considered a reading problem, being described by her teacher as "fairly good." Her problem was a total lack of number concept. In addition she was unable to copy correctly from the board.

Her verbal IQ tested at 90 and her performance at 80, for a full scale of 84, but other psychological tests indicated this figure might be somewhat low. On the Goodenough Draw-A-Man Test her IQ was indicated at 108.

Neurologically, her difficulties were not notable. Her Bender-Gestalt renderings were only slightly below normal for her age. There were no motor disturbances and no impairment of directional sense or body image. She did, however, have the dysgraphia and dyscalculia of Gerstmann's syndrome. The dysgraphia is shown in Illustrations 36 and 37.

In Illustration 36 she was practicing some spelling words: *before, lesson, ago, rabbit, kitten,* and *dinner.* This was pure copying. It may be seen that on the word *before* she became consistently worse each time she wrote it. *Lesson* was misspelled the first two times; *rabbit* went from worse to impossible; and *dinner* progressed from that to *dinmer.* In Illustration 37, her efforts at a composition are reproduced, along with corrections penned by her teacher. All of this fits the patterns of a dysgraphia.

C.Y.'s dyscalculia was another matter. Her intelligent and interested mother admitted that she had not taken her daughter's mathematical incapacity seriously because she, too, had always had difficulty calculating and considered her child merely a

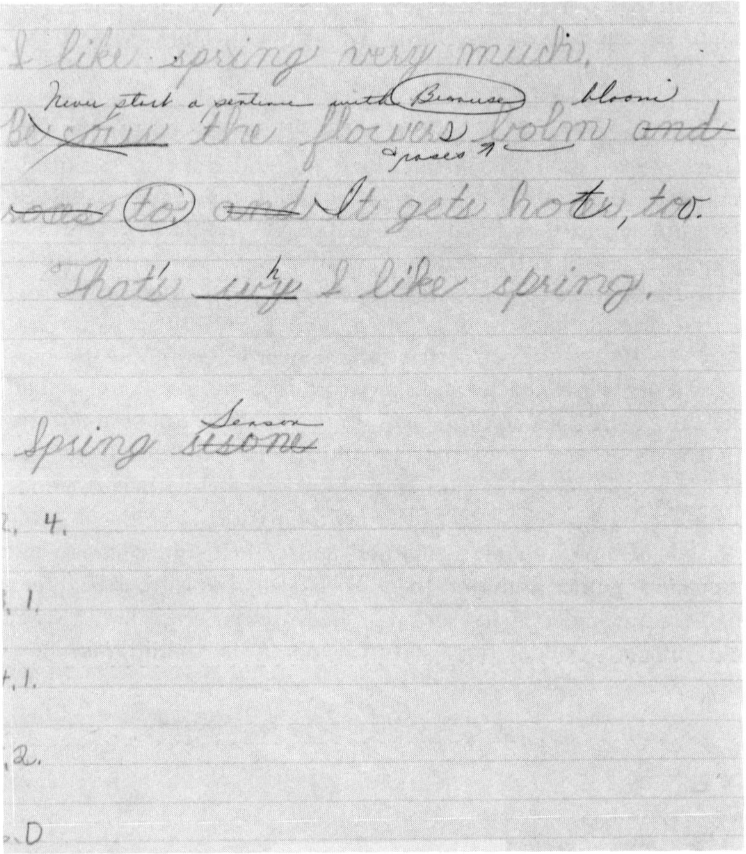

Illustration 37

carbon copy of herself. Thus, the dyscalculia appeared to be familial in origin.

In an effort to improve the patient's abysmal arithmetic, a private tutor was employed. Her report submitted three months after C.Y.'s neurological examination was most revealing, both of good tutoring and the results it can obtain:

"C.Y. started with me March 29. I found her to be a warm friendly child. She was a little shy, but we soon began our work. After she had made several mistakes which upset her slightly (we played a game), we both worked several examples, then checked each other's work. When she found several mistakes in my work, she laughed and said, 'Even you make mistakes.' She enjoys doing work this way. While it appears she is only working five examples, she is actually doing ten in checking my work.

"In addition problems, she will sometimes add one column and subtract one column. When we first started working, she seemed to need me by her side and would ask me every number before she would write it down. She now works very well alone. I made a minus sign in a group of addition problems and she picked this up right away and did the work according to the sign. She is able to put the two and three multiplication tables on the board out of order ($2 \times 7 =$ and $2 \times 3 =$ etc.). She knows these tables and seldom gets mixed up. However, with the four table, she will have the correct combinations (4, 8, 12, etc.) but will write them down incorrectly ($4 \times 12 = 12$ and $4 \times 8 = 44$). In the addition facts, she remembers the even numbers ($6 + 6$, etc.) and is now able to think if $6 + 6 = 12$, then $6 + 7 = 13$. She does not seem to be able to go backwards: $7 + 7 = 14$, therefore $6 + 7 = 13$. She is able to give most answers to the flash cards in order. If the numbers come up in the opposite order, she will sort through the cards until she finds it (for example $\frac{7}{8}$ and $\frac{8}{7}$). She then knows the answer. She does the same with work on the board."

This was progress. The child was fortunate to have good parents and good teachers.

The children we have described have multiple difficulties requiring highly individualized therapy. The common denominator of all is visual imperception. Teaching them to read through phonics and drill in differentiating letters is of paramount importance. If the child has finger agnosia, it seems unlikely that kinesthetic approaches will be very productive. The left-right disorientation poses problems in his pattern recognition and his remedial-reading teacher should be cognizant of his difficulty. But it is not a serious bar to his learning to read.

As for dyscalculia, frankly little is known about teaching methods beyond patience, understanding, and a great deal of drill in basic number facts. It seems likely that the dyscalculic child should be spared all but the most elementary arithmetic. His learning to read is of far greater importance.

I 2.

Visual Imperception with Motor Disability

THE CHILD with perceptual difficulties frequently also has motor problems, as has been indicated in many of the cases presented thus far. The word "motor," in the neurological sense, means "movement." The impaired children of whom we speak do not have normal movement for reasons that are neurological, not muscular.

There are many forms of motor dysfunction, some quite severe. The polio victim, for example, has had a neurological disease which has seriously inhibited his ability to use his limbs. The individual suffering from multiple sclerosis has a neurological disease which grossly affects his motor ability, as does the so-called "cerebral-palsy" patient.

Such severe disorders are familiar to everyone because the motor dysfunction is obvious. But there are a great number of minor motor dysfunctions which, while causing problems for the patient, are not obvious to the layman. The child may have difficulty doing repetitive motions, performing independent tasks with each hand, following movements that involve a pattern, and he may be poorly coordinated. There are two common varieties of disordered coordination. One might be illustrated by the drunk. He is definitely uncoordinated in using his limbs to walk, for example, or reaching out for another drink. He is unsteady and his balance is lamentable, making him "tipsy." Another type of uncoordination, and it is this to which we refer, involves the use of the extremities in repetitive, patterned maneuvers.

We test for neurological motor difficulty in several ways, some of which can be described. In one test, the patient sits in a chair and places his hands on his thighs, palms down. Then he is asked to turn one hand over so that the palm is up and then down. He is made to repeat this alternative pronation and supination as rapidly and accurately as possible. He is asked to do this with one hand and then with the other and then with both hands. This is done with the hands in similar positions and in opposite positions, so that one is pronated while the other is supinated.

The child with motor difficulty may have several problems in performing this. In order to move the hand from a palms-down, or pronated, position to a supinated position, the right hand must be moved clockwise and the left hand counterclockwise. The child may start out doing this and then, as he endeavors to pick up speed, become confused about the pattern and try to move in the opposite fashion, becoming thoroughly frustrated. He may perform properly with one hand but not with the other, so that when he attempts to follow the pattern with both hands making opposite motions, he gives up in confusion. Or, he may perform the motions accurately but be extremely slow, as though concentrating on each movement. The normal child of school age performs these movements quite easily.

Another quite common peculiarity which manifests itself with this test is "mirror motion." When the patient is pronating and supinating with one hand, the other hand moves involuntarily. He can keep it still only with effort, if he is aware of this mirror motion.* It moves back and forth in imitation of the other hand. Occasionally this mirroring is so exaggerated that it is difficult to tell which hand is supposed to be moving! Mirroring is usually a dysfunction associated with the hyperactive child, the youngster who squirms and jumps and can't sit still, and who also is highly distractible and has an abnormally short attention span.

The test just described involves patterned repetition of one motion. Another test seeks to determine the ability of a child to do independent motion with each hand on the order of rubbing the abdomen and patting the head. We use a less familiar but more measurable test. While having him open and close one hand as rapidly as possible, we have him make a tight fist with the other. The tester places *two* of his own fingers in this fist so that any mirroring of the open-close routine from the opposite side may be felt. This procedure is then repeated reversing the hands.

* We have seen patients, when they become aware of the mirroring of one hand, go to the extreme of sitting on the offending member to keep it still!

A normal child will do this simple exercise easily, but the patient with neurological motor difficulties will have several problems. His motion may be slow or irregular or confused, or he may be totally unable to perform it. He may stop or hesitate and forget what he is supposed to be doing and begin some entirely different exercise.

Another test of motor praxis is tandem walking. The patient is shown a straight line on the floor and asked to walk along it so that the heel of the preceding foot touches the toe of the antecedent foot. There should be no space between the feet.

A normal person does this quite expertly. But in the impaired child, a number of problems occur. His balance may be faulty, so that he cannot refrain from moving his arms—and some just have to hold onto the wall. He may move both arms, in the manner of a tightrope walker, or only one arm. It may be the arm on the side opposite to the foot he is moving or, most interestingly, the arm on the same side as the foot.*

A patient may become very disorganized performing this exercise. He'll place one foot in front of the other all right, and then be unable to figure out which foot he is supposed to move next. Is it the back foot? Or the forward foot? This indecision can be observed. Sometimes the child will incorrectly decide it must be the forward foot. He'll slide the forward foot and then move the back foot up to meet it. Occasionally the child will place one foot in front of the other properly and correctly move the back foot forward. But he'll leave a space. This will puzzle him, for he knows this space isn't supposed to be there. But he's not sure how to remedy it. He may slide the front foot back or he may decide the way out of the difficulty is to slide the rear foot forward to close the space. There are many, many distortions of this exercise, including the child who gets so tied in knots he falls in a heap on the floor.

These exercises, as well as others, are indicators of motor apraxia,[1] that is, the inability to execute purposeful patterned movements. The diagnosis is important in reading disorders because it indicates the extent of the child's neurological involvement. The areas of the brain controlling such physical motions are thought to be in close proximity to those areas governing

---

* This has no relationship to a tonic neck reflex.

perceptual processes so it is not uncommon to find that the child with impaired perception also has one or more motor problems.

These motor difficulties have an application to school performance. The physical-education teacher most definitely ought to be interested in them. The classroom teacher should, too. Handwriting certainly involves execution of purposeful repetitive motion and is far more precise than pronating and supinating the hand or walking a crack in the floor.

Use of pattern is integral to many school functions. In reading, the child is repetitiously following patterns of sound, of spelling, of syntax. In arithmetic, addition and subtraction, multiplication and division form patterns which pose problems for a significant number of children.

Diagnosis of motor apraxia should be helpful to parents who fail to understand and frequently carp at their offspring because they don't tie shoelaces; or, when setting the table, put out the silverware in a pattern resembling total chaos; or who are haphazard and disorganized, easily distracted and "forgetful" of what they are supposed to be doing. All children, particularly males, are sloppy and uncoordinated and less than interested in repetitious chores, but for some children the highest motivation and the direst threats of parental discipline will not aid their performance. Almost uniformly, parents of patients with motor apraxia have been relieved to know the nature of the child's difficulty. They have new understanding and sympathy and can help the child cope with his really quite minor limitations.

This parental and teacher understanding is important because, quite often, motor difficulties are maturational. The limitations of motion improve with age, frequently disappearing altogether. There should be no psychological scars left either.

Case No. 15. N.M. was a nine-and-a-half-year-old girl in the fourth grade. She was bright and alert, as evidenced by her WISC test, which showed a verbal IQ of 106, a depressed performance IQ of 96, for a full scale of 101. The individual WISC tests showed she was above average in information, comprehension, similarities, vocabulary, and picture arrangement, but below average in arithmetic, picture completion, block design, and coding, and educable-retarded in object assembly.

The psychologist who tested her made the following observations: "She has a habit of constantly moving her feet. She is generally restless at all times. She is emotionally insecure and immature. She is quite high-strung. If she does not get her own way, she has tantrums. She has difficulty keeping her mind on her work." Her school performance showed "great difficulty" in reading and all related subjects and she was due to fail the fourth grade. The psychologist reported, "On the Wide Range Achievement Test her spelling was so bizarre as to appear organically caused. She cannot copy from the blackboard. Her mother says she cries over the large amount of homework." Her teacher felt the patient knew her work but could not put it on paper.

N.M. had a severe problem in visual perception, particularly with spatial relationships. She found it necessary to turn either the paper or her body to complete the Bender-Gestalt figures.

Neurological examination indicated a number of small peculiarities. There was a maternal history of left-handedness, yet she was right-handed. The nails of her left thumb and great toe were larger than those on the right, indicating perhaps some disorder of dominance. She did repetitive motion and independent motion poorly with both hands, but was better on her right than her left side. In sharp contrast, her tactile perception was markedly better on her left than her right, both in testing graphesthesia and stereognostic ability.

This patient, then, had perceptual difficulties together with disorganized motion. Considering all these problems, she was doing rather well, reading only a year below her grade level. But it seemed that the physical demands of school performance were too much. It took so long for her to perform tasks, physical and intellectual, because of her handicaps, that what must have seemed a mountain of homework became rather terrifying. Lessening of the load upon her and granting her more time in which to perform tasks, while transferring her to a school where she could receive careful remedial reading, were indicated.

Case No. 16. J.B. was an eight-year-old boy in the second grade. He read at the low first-grade level and tended to reverse letters. He frequently spelled *run* as *unr* or sometimes made the *r* in *run* backwards. He always reversed *b* and *d*. His Bender-Gestalt drawings were startling, showing marked deficit in spatial relationship, as in Illustration 38.

The most interesting thing about this patient was his handedness. He was consistently right-handed in all his activity, yet he had a pronounced family history of left-handedness, with two sinistral brothers. The nails of his left thumb and great toe were noticeably larger.

The superiority of his left hand over his chosen right hand showed in many ways. His tactile perception was better on the left than the right in testing for both graphesthesia and stereognostic ability. Interestingly, in the latter test when he was asked to identify an object with his eyes closed, he could identify it with his right hand, but if allowed to do so, he would shift the object to his left hand to make the identification.

His motor ability was satisfactory in either hand, but it was better on the left than on the right. His repetitive motion was quite slow and he confused the pattern, especially when doing independent motion. But he was somewhat better at independent motion when called upon to open and close his left hand than vice versa. His tandem walking was slow and disorganized. He had great difficulty staying on the straight line.

Why did this young man choose his right hand when his left was obviously so superior? No definitive answer can be given, but possibly the same dysfunction which impaired his perception also necessitated a shift in handedness. He was young. One could hope that he would become an average reader—in time, but only with a lot of help.

Case No. 17. H.D. was an eight-year-old boy in the process of failing the first grade for the second time. He had such severe problems that he could not even come close to spelling his own name, and it was a simple one. His IQ by the Stanford-Binet test had been 80 a year before. The WISC produced a different result. His verbal IQ was 96 and his performance IQ 85, for a full scale of 91. The only performance test above the mentally-retarded level was in coding.

His visual perception was quite terrible, as indicated by the Bender-Gestalt drawing in Illustration 39. (Note grouping of most figures on the left half of the page.)

It was his motor performance that was most revealing, however. In doing repetitive motion he started off with a good pattern, but in a few seconds the pattern deteriorated, and soon

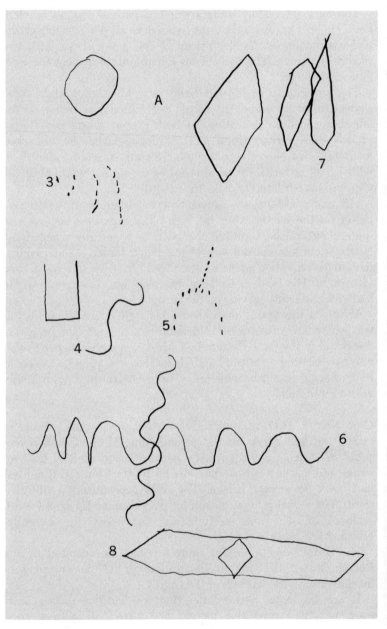

Illustration 38

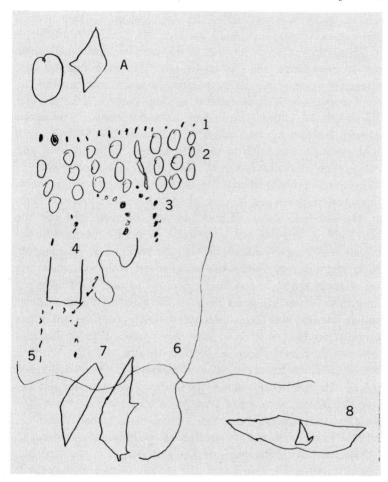

Illustration 39

he was doing something entirely different than he had been instructed to do. There was a little mirror motion, too. He had absolutely no ability to do independent motion. He understood what he was to do, and he tried as hard as he could, but it was just impossible. One could not help but wonder how often his parents and teachers had accused him of not following directions or not paying attention in manual tasks. He suffered not from unwillingness or inattention in this area, but from total incapacity.

Next, H.D. was instructed to do tandem walking and a demonstration was performed for him. He nodded his head in understanding of what he was to do—and promptly walked on *two* straight lines, one for each foot. He was stopped and instructed again. His full cooperation was enlisted and he listened attentively. Now he tried it and did quite well for the first four steps. Then the pattern began to deteriorate. The space between his feet became wider, and by the time he had taken eight steps he was back to walking on two different lines and finally on no particular line at all. He was just going for a stroll.

The patient obviously had a deficiency in pattern memory, which was shown when he was asked to take his shoes and socks off. He had both shoes off and had one sock removed and the other half off when he was distracted. When he returned to the task, he could not remember whether the sock was to go on or off. His frustration was observable as he toyed with both removing and donning the sock, and finally decided to take it off. When it came time to put his shoes back on, he delayed the process as long as possible and finally proceeded slowly, until he got to the second shoe. He put it on at least three times, slipping his heel back out as though he were having trouble. Finally, when it came time to tie his shoes, it was obvious why he had delayed so long. He was totally unable to tie his shoelaces and did not have the faintest concept of how to go about it. He crossed the laces and that was it. The patient's father said he had shown his son how to tie laces many times, but he could never remember it.

Discussion with the boy's father revealed that the boy had difficulty with arithmetic, but it was usually written arithmetic. If given verbal problems, he did them fairly well, although he had little concept of the numbers or philosophy behind them. He didn't know, for instance, what 16 meant, although he was able to add a digit to or subtract one from 16. If called upon to write this result, however, he was unable to do it, producing 61, perhaps, or 19.

At the time he was examined, it was felt that this patient was the case of the year. He not only had perceptual and motor limitation, but he had severe problems in pattern memory. His crude memory in the present was satisfactory, and he was learning to read a little—and it would improve with phonics. The difficulties to be surmounted were quite sizable, nonetheless.

Case No. 18. W.A. was a nine-year-old boy in the second grade who produced some notable renderings of the Bender-Gestalt figures, as shown in Illustration 40.

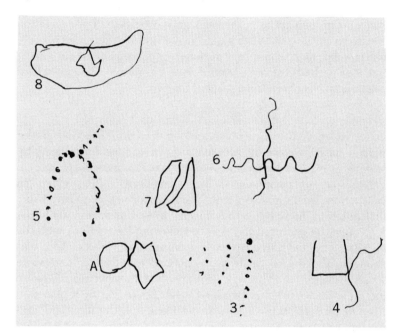

Illustration 40

This result stemmed both from his poor visual perception and his rather considerable motor difficulties.

He, too, had a handedness problem. He was left-handed in almost everything he did, as was his father. However, the right thumbnail was larger, but the left toenail was larger. This was in contrast with the father, whose handedness is confirmed by his nail size. The patient was inaccurate with the movements of his left hand, compared to those of the right. When asked to touch his nose with his left hand, for example, he missed the target quite consistently.

He had difficulty performing motion of any variety. He was

unable to pronate and supinate even one hand successfully, and to perform this maneuver with both hands or to do independent motion was out of the question. If anything, he was worse at it with his chosen left hand than with his right.

This patient was already psychically defeated by his scholastic and physical failures, so he was spared many tests which might have been performed. Enough had been found in any event. He had severe perceptual problems and difficulty in his cerebral cortex on both sides. This would make both reading and writing difficult for him. Some maturational improvement might occur, but it was doubtful if he would ever be normal. Special school placement was absolutely essential for him.

Case No. 19. V.B. was a seven-and-a-half-year-old second-grader with a most fascinating problem, which can be introduced by looking at his Bender-Gestalt drawings in Illustrations 41 and 42.

This patient perseverated on instructions. When given an instruction, he understood it well and performed properly. From that point on, however, unless specific alteration was made in the technique, he confused the next or following instructions with the previous one and came up with a mixed performance. This was shown in Illustration 41. It was explained to him that there were seven drawings that he was to make, that they would all go on the same sheet. The first Bender-Gestalt figure was then placed in front of him. He drew figure A, the circle and the diamond, and started to draw it again. He was stopped and we scratched through the second circle and presented him with the third figure. He took one look at this and drew seven circles and stopped. Then, presented with the fourth Bender-Gestalt figure, he drew seven U-shaped figures without the curved piece being attached. All of this shows on Illustration 41.

At this point, he was stopped and given new instructions that he was to draw figure 3 again, draw it once just the way it appeared on the card, and when he had finished he was to stop. In this manner, with patient individualized instruction on each figure, he managed the renderings which appear in Illustration 42.

As can be seen, these drawings weren't very good. He had problems in visual perception, which were grossly compounded by his most unusual tendency to perseverate on instructions.

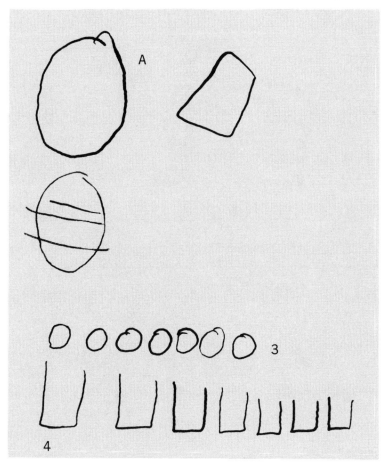

Illustration 41

Another example of this was apparent when he attempted tandem walking. He was told to walk along a crack on the floor. He did so, but balanced himself by holding onto the wall. In order to prevent this and obtain an idea of what his balance was like, he was asked to move out to the next crack in the floor, about seven inches away. At this point he would be unable to reach the wall. His reaction to the instruction was to put one foot on one line and the other foot on the second line in such a way that he was so constricted that movement was totally impossible. When an

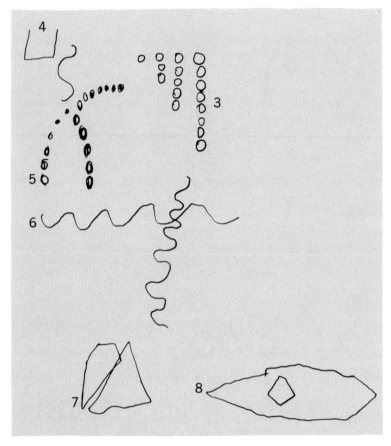

Illustration 42

effort was made to straighten out this impasse with oral instruction, his foot and leg position became even more confused.

At this point we whistled, clapped our hands and disturbed his balance so both feet came off both lines. He was then given a new set of most explicit instructions in tandem walking. He then performed admirably.

From a neurological standpoint, this case was a real "head scratcher." The cause of this child's perseveration was at best elusive. One could have sympathy, however, for the teacher attempting to instruct him in the classroom. A great deal of time and patience would be needed with this fellow. He would be able to learn, but it would not be easy to teach him.*

Case No. 20. A.D. was a six-and-a-half-year-old girl whose verbal performance in school was satisfactory, but when asked to put anything in writing, the result was less than ideal. One of the reasons for this showed in the Bender-Gestalt renderings in Illustration 43.

These drawings—and her signature, which cannot be reproduced here, was even more revealing—indicated both perceptual and motor problems. She did not perceive the figures well, but in addition to this, she had two types of motor difficulty. First, there was a cerebellar problem which made her hand shake so that the pencil moved erratically on the paper. This showed, too, when her hand shook as she endeavored to touch her nose and in the unsteadiness with which she sought to do tandem walking. On top of this, she had a cerebral problem in motion. She was able to do repetitive motion only very slowly and her pattern was poor. Her ability to do independent motion was quite unsatisfactory.

This conglomeration of problems posed great difficulty for her in school. Because of her poor cerebellar and cerebral motion, she

* The perseveration demonstrated by this young man is similar in many ways to that recently attributed to frontal-lobe injury.[2]

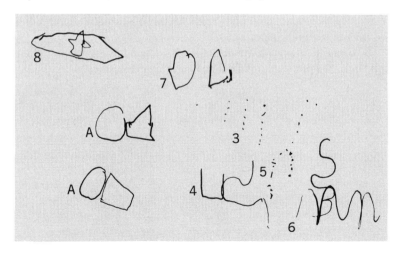

Illustration 43

wrote and drew poorly, and because she had impaired visual perception, she was unable to realize just how poorly she was doing. In other words, her visual imperception kept her from having control over her movements. She was young. There was reason to believe her cerebellar problems would improve in time. Meanwhile she was in great need of understanding, both in school and at home, of her manual limitations.

At this point we would like to present an example of a child who has a problem in motion without perceptual difficulties. The material presented in Illustration 44 is a spelling paper from a fifth-grader of quite high intelligence, who had an intention tremor which was cerebellar in origin. It can be seen that he spelled reasonably well, but he wrote like an "old man," a factor which hopefully his teachers took into consideration. The nature of this child's tremor was such that it occurred when he consciously set out to do fine motor work, such as writing. In any other gross physical activity he performed well.

The motor disabilities which have been the focus of this chapter pose relatively little difficulty for the remedial-reading teacher. The diagnosis of motor problems is important if it indicates the child is weak in following a pattern—a most important aspect of reading. He needs work in recognizing and following the patterns of written language. The diagnosis of motor difficulty will also rule out some of the kinesthetic approaches requiring manual dexterity.

But again, the primary difficulty is visual imperception. Therapy calls for phonics and drill in letter discrimination.

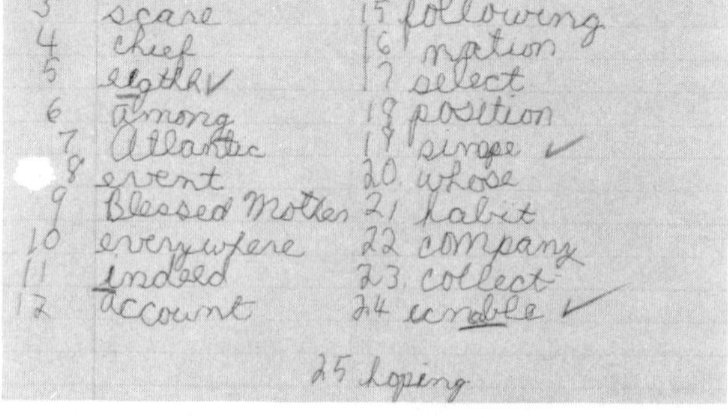
1 juice
2 heaven
3 scare
4 chief
5 eigthrV
6 among
7 Atlantic
8 event
9 Blessed Mother
10 everywhere
11 indeed
12 account
13 language
14 artist
15 following
16 nation
17 select
18 position
19 singee
20 whose
21 habit
22 company
23 collect
24 enable
25 hoping

Illustration 44

13.

Auditory Imperception

VISUAL IMPERCEPTION, which has been discussed and illustrated thus far, makes reading difficult for those so impaired. The child fails at the first task in reading—discriminating the graphic symbols on paper. He cannot distinguish, certainly as precisely as he must, the shapes of the letters in the alphabet.

If, in addition to that, he has impaired tactile perception, another pathway into language comprehension (see Illustration 1) is blocked. If he also has poor motor ability, he may have difficulty writing the letters and this means of learning the shapes of the letters is further hobbled. He may have a disorganized sense of pattern, which may disrupt the entire sequence of reading and spelling. In the case histories presented, we have attempted to show that there are children (and by presenting a lot of cases we are trying to intimate that there are many youngsters) who have severe and multiple disabilities.

As difficult as these cases are, however, they pale before the child who has auditory imperception. He cannot read, that is, he cannot translate marks on paper into sound, because he does not correctly hear the sounds.* If his impairment is more severe, he cannot even approach the task of learning to read. Because he hears sounds incorrectly, he cannot even speak correctly.

Fortunately, auditory imperception seems to be considerably less common than visual imperception. At least in our practice,

---

* We are referring here to those children with a mild to moderate degree of impairment, of course. Those children with severe auditory imperception or congenital sensory aphasia,[1] may never speak sufficiently to be introduced to formal education.

we have encountered far fewer cases of it, because we examine children from a regular school system primarily.

In diagnosing auditory imperception, psychologists commonly administer the "Wepman Test,"[2] in which the child picks out words by the different sounds they make. Ordinarily, the auditory imperception can be detected by the patient's speech. By listening carefully, it is possible to identify sounds the child hears incorrectly.

This speech defect has no relationship to a dysarthria, or disorder of articulation, which a speech therapist treats, such as a lisp, stutter, poor enunciation, improper formation of sounds, and other defects. The child with auditory imperception may or may not have a dysarthria, but if he does, it is coincidental. The hearing imperception causes the child to make improper substitutions of sounds. He may enunciate them clearly, but often, in an effort to hide his peculiar speech (he knows it from the reactions of others), he has developed slurs and other speech patterns—or has cultivated the art of silence.

In a neurological examination, we listen to the child's spontaneous speech and, when necessary, get him to say certain test phrases. In addition, we seek to learn the history of his speech development. How early did he talk in words and sentences? Has he had any problems or been in speech therapy?

Happily, educators are aware of the relationship between disordered speech and disordered reading. Speech therapy begins in the first grade in most modern schools. It may be said that the child with auditory imperception has a greater chance of being helped than the student whose problem is visual or motor. But as the following cases illustrate, this is not always so.

Case No. 21. R.M. was a boy, five years and ten months old, who had been having difficulty in kindergarten. Part of his problem was emotional immaturity. His mother had been hospitalized for protracted periods and he was cared for by a number of relatives who doted on him and waited on him hand and foot. The effect of this was to make his borderline intelligence less useful to him and to exaggerate his neurological difficulties.

In kindergarten he received speech therapy, but it was stopped because he had made no progress. He also failed an eye test, the question being raised whether this was due to a disorder of vision or because of low intelligence.

The patient's immaturity and unwillingness to cooperate made neurological testing difficult. He seemed to have unusual eye motion as his eyes did not converge on a near object. Whether this was neurological or optic could not be determined. He had some tremor of his hands on any voluntarily performed motion and there was gross discoordination of repetitive motion. His pattern of motion was quite poor.

Most striking was his speech disorder. Some of it was infantile and could be considered to be emotional but some of it was organic. For example, he substituted consonants in a way which bore no resemblance to an emotional speech disorder. This first showed itself when he was asked what he did in kindergarten. He replied, "Oh, *hingerfaint.*" Asked what that was, he said, "You know what hingerfainting is. You smear haint." Asked if he meant *fingerpaint,* he said, with a tinge of annoyance at the examiner's obtuseness, "That's it, *hingerfaint.*"

Some effort was expended to get this patient to say *fingerpaint* again in a natural context. It was ultimately accomplished, only this time he said *pingerfaint,* reversing the consonants of the first and third syllables. He frequently substituted h and p and also was heard to substitute an f for the c in *crayon,* among others. He did not correctly perceive the sounds of certain consonants—auditory imperception.

By itself, his condition was not incorrectable at his age. What was discouraging about this case, though, was his low intelligence coupled with gross mishandling at home. His parents appeared to have no understanding of his problem after it was explained to them. Recommendation was made to have the child repeat kindergarten. It would at least keep him away from his relatives for several hours a day, while exposing him to the organized activity and patterned performance which he needed. And at the same time the school was to work with his speech, slowly and patiently.

Case No. 22. C.J. was a ten-year-old tragedy. She sat in the office, cowering. She slumped in her chair, face down, hands on lap, pulling at the fabric of her dress. She was unresponsive and reticent to the point of total uncommunication.

She was the product of a good home. Her mother spoke of her anxiety and concern for her daughter and of her willingness to do anything to help her.

She needed it. For the last three years this child had been installed in classes for educable-retarded children, partly on the basis of a WISC which showed a verbal IQ of 66, a performance IQ of 86 for a full scale of 73. Another reason was that no one had succeeded in teaching her anything. Now she was so withdrawn and fearful of new experiences that educational efforts were quite frustrated. At age ten, she could count to 13 and write her first name. In contrast she was able to swim well and to ride a bicycle, along with other physical activities.

Eighteen months previously, when the child was eight and a half, she had spent several days at a clinic where she had been probed, prodded and diagnosed in almost every conceivable way. Included in the study was an electroencephalogram, skull X rays, blood count, routine urinalysis, tests for PKU, thyroid function and tuberculosis, a complete set of measurements of the body and the head, chest, abdomen, plus a routine physical examination. Neurological examination was said to be difficult because of her anxiety, but otherwise normal. She was then seen by a psychologist, speech pathologist and an audiologist. In the summary of this study (12 typewritten pages) the pediatrician states: "There is no question that she is functioning at a subnormal intellectual level within the borderline range of intelligence. There is evidence of central-nervous-system impairment as measured by the neurological examination (said in the report to be normal), psychological testing, speech and language evaluation, behavior pattern and abnormal electroencephalogram. Her greatest problem is undoubtedly subnormal intellectual functioning in association with uneven abilities consistent with organicity. . . . Speech and language evaluation indicates she has a mild articulation problem as well as generally reduced language skills. Comprehension, auditory retention, recall of digits, auditory discrimination, verbal expressive skills and conceptualization are impaired. Audiometric testing reveals good auditory acuity."

She was then returned to the same school placement, only on medication because of the abnormalities seen on her electroencephalogram.

Despite her fears and unwillingness—her reaction to every

overture was that she couldn't possibly do it—some testing was performed. She had a gross problem in visual perception as may be seen in Illustration 45.

In contrast, her tactile perception was surprisingly good. She also had some motor problems, doing repetitive patterns slowly and with great difficulty. She was unable to do independent motion.

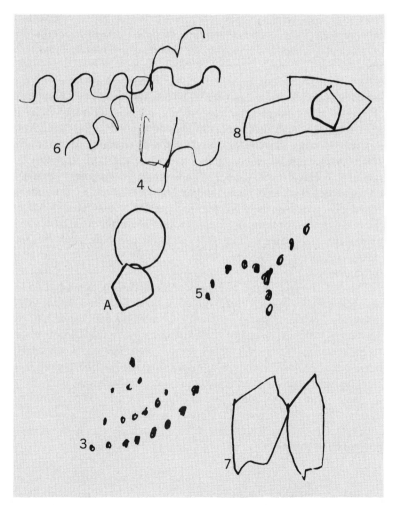

Illustration 45

All of this testing was performed in silence. We almost despaired of getting her to speak. Several conversational entries were tried, but to no avail. Finally, she was asked to name her favorite television program. She replied, so softly it was almost inaudible, "*Fatman*." When we said we were not acquainted with that program, she said, "You know, the guy who looks like a *fat* and has that little boy with him."

This was auditory imperception. She sat before the family television and heard *fat* for *bat*. She presumably played with a *fat* and *fall*. There were a number of other substitutions in the few words she spoke, including the fact that she was her mother's *darter*.

This child was not retarded in the accepted meaning of the word. She had a gross disorder of visual and auditory perception at age ten. One could only imagine how disordered it had been at ages four, five and six. Certainly, her continued failure to differentiate certain consonant sounds was a residual of a severe auditory-perceptual difficulty at an earlier age. This inability to perceive correctly the sounds which others uttered left her with an informational and thus an intellectual deficit. Conversation could not possibly have made much sense to her and her own distorted reproductions of those sounds must have been incomprehensible to others. The confusion, frustration, ridicule led surely to silence. No one could possibly guess at her true intelligence.

This child had a long way back. The first step appeared to be an attack upon her auditory imperception. This had to be done primarily by the parents, patiently correcting misstatement, repeating as often as necessary the correct sounds until she learned to discriminate them and to say them. Then, her excellent tactile perception offered a means to reinforce her visual perception. Feeling and drawing letters and shapes provided a way in to language comprehension. Time and patience and effort would be needed, but there was at least a possibility of success. The ultimate tragedy was that the school in which she was enrolled had no such program.

The therapy for the child with auditory imperception will be obvious to readers by this time. He will best learn to read through visual and kinesthetic means. This is the one neurologically impaired child for whom the look-say method is an advantage. But it must be said that even a slight auditory imperception is so debilitating that relatively little progress can be made until the child correctly learns to differentiate sounds. Here is where primary emphasis must be placed by patiently pointing out the child's errors and insisting that he correct them.

14.

Specific Dyslexia

THERE ARE MANY strange neurological disorders simply because of the complexity and resourcefulness of the human brain. In this category are a group of dyslexia cases, children who have a pronounced reading disability that has no apparent neurological cause. These cases are customarily called *specific* or *familial* or *primary dyslexia*.

Neurologists shy away from talking about specific dyslexia for the simple reason that no physician likes to talk about a condition he can't explain—or at least hypothesize about. These are uncanny cases, apparently normal youngsters who pass every neurological test, yet who have reading disorders. On examination one finds no disorder of visual, tactile or auditory perception, no motor disability of any kind, no speech defect, no neurological dysfunction in conjunction with or in explanation of the failure to read. Some authorities have suggested that, if the examiner looks long enough and hard enough, he will find something. But every neurologist has had cases that defied this effort.

An illustration of this was a patient referred by his father, a rather prominent professional man. The boy, a ninth-grader in an exclusive private school, had always had a reading problem despite extensive remedial-reading instruction. This had been quite beneficial, bringing him up to the fifth-grade reading level, but all efforts to improve his reading further had failed. He was a fine boy with superior intelligence, an engaging personality and great athletic skill.

Exhaustive neurological examination of him was entirely fruitless. If there had ever been a neurological explanation for his disorder, it had long since disappeared. His visual perception, for example, was satisfactory, yet the fact remained that he read only slowly and inaccurately and spelled the same way. The only available diagnosis was that this young man had a fairly mild case of specific dyslexia. It was suggested to the patient and his father that the remedial reading and the pressure to better his reading performance be stopped. The boy read about as well as he was ever going to and remedial instruction was distracting and, frankly, a waste of time.

The patient's reaction was one of relief. "This is what I've been trying to tell everyone for years," he said. He had long since accepted the fact that he was a poor reader, that he would have to work longer and harder than other people, that he would not enter an occupation that required a great deal of rapid reading. He accepted disability with the same equanimity that he accepts the fact he has blue eyes—a most admirable attitude. In the months that followed, improvement in both his academic and athletic skills was noted, attributable to his more relaxed and confident attitude.

What is most interesting about this case is that the father revealed that he, too, had always been a poor reader. "I never admitted it to anyone, but I was a terrible reader. I was sort of the dunce in the family and entered my profession because my family expected me to. Fortunately, I've worked it out so I can read as little as possible."

Then, he asked if he could use the phone, saying, "I've just got to tell my sister." It seems that his sister, a woman of national prominence, had always been smarter and more erudite than her brother. Now on the phone with her, he said, with the greatest delight, "Hey, sis, I just found out why *your* son can't read."

This father's admission and phone call confirmed the diagnosis, for the one fact that enables a physician to diagnose specific dyslexia is that it is familial. Specific dyslexia may occur as an acquired rather than as a genetic condition (personally, we can see no reason that it should not!), but I don't think any neurologist is brave enough to make a diagnosis without some supporting evidence.

Neurologists are not very comfortable when discussing specific dyslexia. Perhaps the best use of the term is to describe cases like the above—persons whose neurological dysfunctions have disappeared, leaving an observable residue only in their reading and writing deficiencies. The suspicion is increasing that specific dyslexia is a rather pretentious neurological euphemism for ignorance. The term has become a catch-all expression for a growing list of neurological dysfunctions. It is to be hoped that its use will end entirely one day soon.

Since the first edition of this book was published in 1968, several neurological dysfunctions leading to learning disabilities have been identified and described. Only a few years ago, youngsters with these disabilities would have been labeled "specific dyslexics." Today we know better. Neurologists are learning, too —from their patients.

The newly identified dysfunctions fall into three groups. The first of these involves what educators call *sound-symbol relationships* and what philologists call *semiosis*—the function of signs and symbols in communication. Three semiotic disorders have been recognized so far. In the simplest of these, the child has difficulty in making the link between a sound and its printed symbol. He may recognize the sound *bah* but be unable to recognize that the letters *ba* make the sound *bah*. To attempt to teach such a child to read through phonics is to invite disaster.

Another semiotic difficulty relates to the sequencing, or ordering, of letters and sounds. The child will jumble sounds and letters, as in "pasghetti" or "hoppity hip." This may be routine and amusing in a four-year-old, but an eight-year-old who does it faces serious problems in reading and writing as well as speech.

Still another semiotic problem, recently identified, has to do with the ability to rearrange or manipulate sounds. In language, all of us are constantly manipulating a rather small supply of sounds so as to form the hundreds of thousands of words in our vocabulary. To give a simple example, a person takes three small sounds to make the word *tap*, rearranges them to form the word *pat*, then rearranges them once more for the word *apt*.

Some children have great difficulty with such manipulation of sounds, as described by Charles H. and Patricia C. Lindamood. They developed a rather simple test to identify the problem.* It uses colors to represent sounds. For example, the sound of *u*

* Lindamood Auditory Conceptualization (L. A. C.) Test (Teaching Resources, Boston, Mass.).

as in *up* might be blue; the sound of *p* as in *pot,* or the terminal sound in *up,* might be green, and the *s* sound might be yellow. Hearing the syllable *ups* (letters are not used), the child should display the colors blue, green, yellow. If the syllable *usp* is uttered, the child should rearrange the colors to blue, yellow, green. A child of eight should be able to do this easily. Failure in the exercise indicates a neurological dysfunction. Learning to read by phonics will be difficult for such a child, and later he will probably encounter problems with arithmetic. The Linda-moods not only designed the test to identify the problem but also devised a training program to help such patients.*

The second of the newly recognized dysfunctions relates to word finding. The child knows the word—it is stored somewhere in his brain, but he cannot find it when he needs it. Everyone has this difficulty some of the time. In fact, we have invented a vocabulary to cover our deficiencies, including such expressions as "thingamajig" or "thingamabob" and "whatchacallit." Where a normal child may have problems in word finding once or twice out of ten times, some children will miss as many as eight times out of ten.

Word-finding difficulties are hard to identify because so many words are judgmental. A person moving rapidly down the street may be said to be walking fast, running or jogging, among other descriptives. Two people in conversation can be talking, chatting, arguing or so forth. The judgmental problem in using adjectives is even more difficult. How many ways are there to describe a sunset?

We have developed a simple test to indicate word-finding problems. The child is shown a series of pictures of objects that have only one name. Some of the simple ones are an ambulance, caboose, fire hydrant. More difficult ones are binoculars, a thermometer, a propeller. The pictures are shown to the child one at a time. The normal child should be able to name the object promptly and accurately. The impaired child will be hesitant, inaccurate and frequently stymied. From years of practice in hiding his problem, such a child may be extremely clever in concealing his word-finding difficulties. An illustration of this is the response of a recent patient asked to identify a caboose. The

* Auditory Discrimination in Depth (Teaching Resources, Boston, Mass.).

following exchange took place:

"What is that?"

The child, after a prolonged hesitation: "That's a—a—it's a train"

Now, the child knew very well it wasn't a train but, unable to think of the word *caboose*, he hoped to get away with *train*. It is important to try to have the child say the precise word.

"It's not the whole train, is it? It's only part of the train. What part is it?"

"It's the—ah—the—you know, the red car at the end."

"That's true, but what do you call it?"

"Well, it's the place where the men who work on the train sleep."

"That's also true, but what do you call it?"

The child had now run out of subterfuges and lapsed into frustrated silence. He was given three choices.

"Is it a candle, a carton or a caboose?"

"Of course, it's a caboose!"

This child was very bright and obviously well informed about cabooses. He simply could not find the word for them—and for many other objects. Sometimes a patient will come close to the word, giving a partial answer. A fire hydrant may be called a "fire thing" or even a "fire extinguisher." Words may be confused, so that an ax, first called a hatchet, may be labeled a "hax." A funnel may be mispronounced as "thunnel" or "frummel," a propeller rendered as "capella."

Such children will get by in normal conversation. They'll fake and substitute so that parents and teachers may be unaware of their word-finding difficulties. Then, when the child is put to reading, these difficulties surface. He knows that the letters *c*, *a* and *t* mean a furry animal that purrs, but the filing system in his brain simply will not produce the word *cat*. We are not now able to test it, but we suspect that such a child also has great difficulty in finding verbs, adjectives and so forth, as well as names of objects. At best his reading will be slow and inaccurate.

Neurologists have also begun to recognize a third group of impaired youngsters. A child with repeated ear infections between the ages of two and five may have suffered an undetected intermittent hearing loss which may later cause multiple and various difficulties in reading. These are the crucial years for the development of vocabulary. If a child does not hear words correctly, he will not speak correctly. Later, when he tries to read, his symbol-and-sound sequencing patterns will be disoriented. With inter-mittent hearing loss, a child's ability to hear goes on and off and he will miss whole words or parts of words, or hear them incor-rectly. The word *puzzle* may be heard, for example, as "zell"; or a motorcyclist may wear "gargles" over his eyes. The child heard garbled language and therefore stored garbled language in his brain.

By the time the child reaches the second grade, all clinical evidence of the hearing loss may have disappeared. Only a med-ical history of ear infections will indicate the root of the trouble. When the child takes care in speaking, reading and writing, he may do fine. But when he is tired or pressured and tries to speed up the communication process, he frequently reverts to the gar-bled versions of words so long stored in his system. Such a child needs speech and language therapy—along with patient and understanding parents and teachers.

The following cases are typical of these disorders.

Case No. 23. T. M., seven years and nine months of age, was experiencing great difficulty in the second grade. His mother reported that "he was a little slow in learning to talk, but not enough to worry anyone." Some question had been raised about his hearing, but tests proved it to be normal.

T. M. had attended kindergarten and the first grade in one school, then transferred to another school, where a reading re-source teacher reported he was reading at only a beginning level. He was said to know very few sight words and only a few consonant sounds—and these only at the beginnings of words. The teacher reported: "He did not seem to understand that sounds and their letter symbols can be put together to form words."

Examination showed T. M. to have some motor difficulties. When alternating pronation and supination of the right hand, he tended to mirror the motions with the left, nondominant hand. He was slow in performing patterned motions. His Bender-Gestalt test was done satisfactorily, though slowly—perhaps another in-dication of motor difficulties. Both his tactile perception and his stereognosis were good for his age. When the L. A. C. test was administered, T. M. did very poorly. He really had no concept of the idea of manipulation of phonemes and didn't seem to understand the answers even when they were given to him.

This patient's motor difficulties should probably disappear in time. He did have, however, serious semiotic disabilities. He seemed to have little understanding of the relationship between a letter and a sound. Even if he could gain this, he would then have difficulty in putting sounds in the proper sequence to form a word. Remediation of this young man's problem was going to be very slow, and he would have to count on further neurological development in the future. Unfortunately, his school had no room for T. M. in its remedial reading classes.

Case No. 24. J. B., eight years and two months old, was having difficulties in the second grade. His mother said he was encountering problems in reading and was beginning to develop a poor self-image as a result.

Questioning revealed that J. B.'s speech was not as clear as that of his siblings, although it had appeared at the same time. In fact, his younger sister spoke more clearly than he did. The boy's father said that he, too, had had speech and language difficulties that had hampered him in school.

Testing revealed J. B. to have some motor dysfunction, in particular some limitation of motion in the upper and lower extremities. His Bender-Gestalt was satisfactory. His tactile perception was fair, being about six months behind what it should be for his age. Stereognostic testing showed that he could identify objects by touch but had great difficulty in naming some of them. He knew a door key, for example, but refused to answer because he couldn't think of the name of it. In testing of his word-finding ability, he was unable to identify by name pictures of the dial on a telephone, a fire hydrant and a traffic light. He mispronounced *propeller* by leaving off the first syllable. He insisted a thermometer was a "temperature." When it was suggested that it really was a thermometer, he agreed and said, "Oh, yes, that tells you what grees it is." In trying to identify the traffic light, he started off by calling it a street light, realized this was incorrect, then said it was a telephone light, then a telephone pole and finally stopped trying. His speech showed gross disorder of articulation, with omission of consonants and syllables. These came anywhere at random in the word. Other words were not spoken in recognizable form.

J. B. needed speech therapy in the worst way. Until his articulation and sequencing of sounds were improved, his progress in reading would be very slow.

Case No. 25. C. V., twelve years and three months old, was finishing his second year in a special school for children with learning disabilities. He was having great difficulty in all subjects, especially reading. His family reported that C. V. was late in talking compared with his siblings. His mother first said that his speech was satisfactory, but when questioned admitted that he had had speech difficulties in the past. He still had some problems —for instance, tending to reverse syllables, so that a grass-cutting instrument, for example, was a "mowerlawn." His mother also reported that he had had frequent and severe ear infections until age five, when he had had a tonsillectomy to correct the problem.

Testing showed C. V. to be right-handed, which was confirmed by comparing relative nail size. He had no motor problems. His stereognosis and finger identification test were normal, as was his left/right discrimination. His tactile perception was questionable: he confused 3 and 8 on his right side, and on his left the 9 and 6, as well as the 5 and 2.

His word finding was poor. On being shown a picture of a telephone dial, he called it the face of a telephone, then said the numbers were used to call up other people, then finally said it was a telephone dial. All of this other information was filler to give him time to come up with the word *dial*. At times he falsely denied he knew a word. When told the word, he insisted he had never heard of it, but in later conversation revealed by references to it that he had indeed known it. He made errors in speech, frequently substituting or omitting consonants. His spelling was likewise garbled—so much so that it was often impossible to tell what word he was trying to spell.

It is likely that C. V. may have had some problems with visual perception at an earlier age, which had cleared up by age twelve. This may have added to his reading difficulties. His most serious neurological problem was his garbled speech, probably caused by an early hearing loss. Speech therapy and drill in language were necessary before improvement in reading could be expected.

A few years ago, all these children might have been labeled specific dyslexics. Today we are fortunately able to make more precise diagnoses. It is to be hoped that in the years ahead we will come to understand many more of these unusual cases.

PART FOUR

SUGGESTIONS FOR THERAPY

15.

An Appeal for Acceptance

"IF YOU TEACH a child the letters of the alphabet and the sounds that they make, he will read." That emphatic statement made in private conversation by one of the nation's foremost authorities on reading instruction was one of the spurs for the study and effort that went into this book. This man, the dean of a leading college of education, refused to believe that there are children who cannot for organic reasons learn either the letters or the sounds they represent—or both.

At the risk of trying the patience of readers, we have presented many cases and attempted to be as specific as possible in illustration of the multitude of neurological impairments that can impede reading instruction. Along with the child's organic difficulties, we have tried to show the failure and frustration of the child, parents and teachers.

We believe that unsuspected, unrecognized, undiagnosed neurological disabilities are a major reason that that "hard core" of disabled readers exists year after year with its attendant emotional and vocational repercussions. We are appealing for acceptance by educators that these neurological disorders exist.

Why hasn't dyslexia been accepted as a cause for reading disorders? The principal reason has been simple lack of information. The physicians studying neurological learning disorders have been rather small in numbers, certainly in comparison to the number researching cancer and heart disease. This is quite proper since no one ever dies of dyslexia. Those who have studied neurological learning disorders have reported their findings primarily in the medical literature. Unless parents or teachers make a specific effort to look for books or articles on the subject in a medical library, they remain largely uninformed even that the disorder exists. This lack of information about dyslexia extends not only to lay and educational literature, but to general medical literature as well. Most medical textbooks, if they mention dyslexia at all, do so in a sentence or paragraph. Thus, most general practitioners, pediatricians and internists are not well informed about the disabilities discussed in this book.

In addition to the lack of information—and the natural tendency to be suspicious of something one has never heard of—a number of prominent educators who have heard of dyslexia have disparaged it. Dr. Donald D. Durrell, professor of education at Boston University and one of the nation's most widely respected authorities on reading disorders, has written:[1]

> Unfortunately, educational techniques for prevention and correction of reading difficulties have been slow in development and acceptance. This left a field open to those who have attempted to "explain" reading difficulties on all sorts of neurological and psychological hypotheses. . . . As we progress in the educational analysis of reading difficulties, it becomes increasingly clear that most of the failures in reading rest upon difficulties and confusions in the learning process. Thus the necessity to seek elaborate psychological causes is considerably diminished.

At another point he wrote:[2]

> The early inability of school people to discover and correct the educational causes of reading difficulties left a field open to other approaches. A great deal of mystery was thrown about "nonreaders" and "specific reading disability" by some psychologists and psychiatrists. Neurologic explanation included such items as "congenital word blindness" caused by "lesions in Broca's convolutions" and "strophosymbolia" or "lack of unilateral brain dominance." The latter condition was used to explain reversal tendencies in reading, such as *was* as *saw*, *on* as *no*, and the confusion of *b, d, p,* and *q.* It is now recognized that these reversals are normal in all beginning reading, and are simply confusions resulting from inadequate perception.*
>
> At one time techniques of reading analysis were filled with tests of general perceptual functions such as "visual and auditory

---

* True, such reversals are normal for the beginning reader. But in the fifth grade? And is "inadequate perception" normal?

memory span," "visual analysis and recognition," and "form-sound-meaning association." These tests included various complicated designs, nonsense syllables and other material which have little meaning or interest to the child. The intent of such tests was to discover faulty associational tracts in the child's brain. However, it has long been recognized that such approaches are not helpful in the analysis of reading difficulty.

We submit that such *incorrect* "recognition" has taken place far too long.

A number of other deprecators could be cited, but we would like to mention only one more, quoting from a book by Charlotte Mergentime, reading coordinator of the School Volunteers of the New York City Board of Education and formerly a faculty member of the New York University Reading Institute, in which she wrote:

> Children who confuse *b* and *d*, read words like *was* for *saw*, or reverse letters, syllables, or words, may show symptoms of mixed lateral dominance, or just poor reading habits. In any case, a diagnosis does not have to be made. Whatever the cause, a few simple exercises described in chapter six will quickly solve the problem.[3]

Such confidence is misplaced. More than a few simple exercises is needed to overcome gross disorders of perception, poor directional sense and body image, dysgraphia, dyscalculia, poor motor performance. If a child of seven cannot distinguish a letter from a number, if a boy of thirteen cannot write his own name correctly, if a girl of ten says her favorite television program is *Fatman*, if a boy of fourteen cannot remember his own telephone number—and all the other cases we have presented thus far—we doubt that a few simple exercises will fix them up "jim dandy."

We would like to reply to the doubters and detractors by presenting four case histories of youngsters who have multiple neurological problems, all of them severe. Helping these youngsters is a challenge to educators, psychologists and physicians.

Case No. 26. T.E. was a nine-and-a-half-year-old girl with every possible cause for reading disorders. She entered the first grade at the age of five years and nine months. She was quite emotionally immature and spent most of the first grade crying. Of necessity, she repeated that grade, then was passed to the second, where she was still unable to read. At this time she was seen by a psychologist, who found that she had a verbal IQ of 96, a startling performance IQ of 121, for a full scale of 109—an intelligent child. The psychologist reported: "The cause of the inefficiency, with functioning average, seems to be largely emotional. While there are signs of distortions in perceptual-motor functioning, these seem particularly affected by emotional factors rather than the perceptual-motor area of the central nervous system." As was shown later, he was considerably in error in his opinion of her neurological problems. In any event, the psychologist recommended remedial reading, but warned that remedial teachers "must not be seduced by her baby ways and particularly her attempts to manipulate. The parents must also be made aware of this youngster's needs for control and growing up."

At this point, the child was transferred to another school, where she failed everything because of her reading. She received remedial-reading instruction an hour a day during the school session, but the results were disappointing.

When the patient came in for examination, she was a pretty, happy child. She was willing and cooperative, a child who wanted to please, as though her agreeableness would make up to her parents and teachers for her nearly total failure to read. She confused letters and reversed the directions of letters, as well as the order of letters in words.

On examination, the child showed evidence of visual and tactile imperception. She was hyperactive, with a short attention span and a great degree of distractibility, all of an organic nature. This, together with her emotional immaturity and the fact that she had attended three schools already and was about to be transferred to a fourth, all of which had different methods of teaching reading, made her reading problem inevitable.

Some medication was prescribed to reduce her hyperactivity and enable her to sit still for instruction. But that was only a start. She badly needed to be stabilized in a school situation. She needed intensive instruction in an effort to improve her visual perception and particularly in phonics to make use of her auditory perception. Then she needed some oral instruction to give her the information she was failing to learn because she could not read.

Case No. 27. B.D. was a girl six years and nine months old who was having trouble in the first grade. The psychologist who tested her reported, "She is presently extremely poor in reading; slow in most areas; tends to repeat things; seems to have a preoccupation with one idea at a time. She stares into space. She is not relaxed during sleep—sleeps with her arms crossed. With other children, she 'tenses-up' and stares. She has a very short attention span. The child bites her nails. She seems quite anxious most of the time. She tends to become preoccupied with one idea at a time and will repeat it over and over. She fears aggressive children and is very timid around peers."

Testing on the Stanford-Binet showed an IQ of 91 and she drew Bender-Gestalt figures that were similar to those of a four-year-old, Illustration 50.

The psychologist also reported the following: "She is an attractive young girl who related with cooperation. She seemed to be giving good attention some of the time. At other times she was distractible, giving some attention to a bracelet and to the wide lacy cuffs on her sleeves. At times, she needed urging to answer. She seemed to prefer the easy tasks. She is a little anxious about success, especially in relation to younger members of the family. She seemed somewhat motivated at times, and at others seemed to need encouragement. She has a very slight speech deviation, involving articulation, specifically the use of *f* and *th*."

On examination, there was some indication of a handedness problem. Her left thumbnail was larger, but she was right-handed. Her repetitive motion was done poorly, both in speed and in pattern, and this was particularly true with the left hand. She mirrored motion excessively on the right side and some on the left. She was entirely unable to do either independent motion with each hand or tandem walking, although she tried very hard.

Her tactile perception was very bad, as indicated in Illustration 17 on page 131. Her visual perception was quite immature as shown in Illustration 46. And she had an auditory imperception, which showed both in her consonant substitutions and in her tendency to appear inattentive. She seemed to have difficulty understanding what was said to her.

This, then, was a child who not only had serious motor problems, but had impairment of all three forms of perception used in reading. How was language comprehension to occur

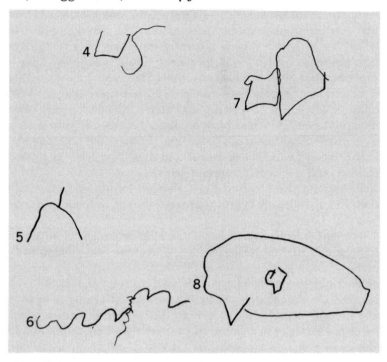

Illustration 46

when she had disorders of visual, auditory and tactile perception? She had the intelligence, but how was she to learn to read? It would not be easy for the schools to teach her, but does that mean the effort should not be made, especially since there was reason to hope that within a few years her perceptual difficulties might improve?

Case No. 28. W.A. was an intelligent eight-year-old boy who had failed the first grade twice. It was not difficult to see why. His testing for oral reading showed he knew precisely two words, *little* and *yellow*. In silent reading he did not know any words. Asked to recognize words on flash cards, he knew one, *me*. Asked to figure out unfamiliar words, he succeeded in reading the word *come*. He was able to identify only a few letters of the alphabet, mistaking *d* for *b*, *y* for *v*, etc. In contrast, he achieved a perfect score in comprehension of third-grade material read to him!

In addition to his obvious impairment of visual perception, he had tactile difficulties of a serious nature. He was unable to identify numbers written on the fingers of the right hand—and he is right-handed—but he did somewhat better but not normally on his left hand. On stereognostic testing, he was able to identify objects by touch, but he had some problem in naming them. It was not as serious as the patient in Case No. 6, but he had a degree of nominal aphasia. In addition, his motion was poor, in pattern, speed and coordination.

This fine young man, then, had visual imperception that virtually eliminated reading and tactile difficulties that hampered that approach to reading instruction. His auditory perception was excellent, but he had a mild aphasia in naming objects. Do schools have a program for him?

Case No. 29. G.N. was a young girl several months past her seventh birthday whose total lack of school performance led her family pediatrician to seek a psychological evaluation. The WISC was administered and showed a verbal IQ of 91, performance IQ of 78, for a full scale of 83. The Bender-Gestalt drawings were on a par with a five-and-a-half-year-old, indicating impaired visual perception. Some of the psychologist's comments provided insight into the child:

"She complied with my instructions and performed all the tasks presented to her, but she had it fixed in her mind that she had come to play with toys, and kept asking: 'How many more? Now can I play with the blocks? What are we going to do next? How long must I stay here?' She stayed put in her chair, but nevertheless she was restless. She smiled a lot, but her smile seemed to be a mere technique, quite unrelated to her feelings. In the verbal part of the WISC she tended to misunderstand instruction; when she misunderstood, she persisted rigidly in her misapprehension. In the performance scale she behaved very unreflectively and gave up very easily in the face of difficulty. She asked for a lot of help, and repeatedly wanted to know: 'Is this right?' If I asked her to tell me if *she* thought it was right, or if I withheld comment, she doubted her own performance. In items which provided a model to copy, she tended to forget about the model and go off on an idea of her own. She gave one response to each of the Rorschach cards and seemed eager to get rid of them. Her Bender-Gestalt performance was pretty chaotic. She took little care with her drawing, and often said, 'I can't do it.' "

The psychologist then summarized: "This is a child who is functioning at a dull-normal level intellectually. Her ego function is very weak. She tries to be compliant, but finds control very difficult. She seems to accept external control fairly cheerfully, and is perhaps threatened by her own inability to control impulse. She tends to be concrete and finds abstraction very difficult. Her visual organization is considerably impaired. Her frustration tolerance is low. She gives up easily in the face of difficulty. There is, on the other hand, capacity for escapist fantasy, and some indication that she has a pretty active inner life—even though it is not too well integrated with what goes on in the world around her. The particular combination of ego weakness, difficulty in control, compliance, restlessness, low frustration tolerance, absence of the truly bizarre, sensuousness, desire to please—together with the concreteness and poor visual organization and the specific Bender pointers—suggest that there is likely to be organic brain damage. There seems more here than emotional immaturity. . . . I therefore recommend neurological examination."

Conversation with the patient's teacher developed that the teacher thought the child had a hearing problem. This was subsequently checked. Her hearing acuity was normal. The teacher also said the child was a management problem in school. She would work briefly, then get up and walk around the room or come up to talk to the teacher. She constantly sought approval from the teacher for any work that she had done or special explanations and instructions.

In addition to visual imperception, the child had impaired auditory perception. She frequently omitted a syllable from a word. This made it extremely difficult to understand what she was saying until one became aware of her speech mechanism. This was why the teacher thought she had a hearing problem. It wasn't her hearing, but her auditory imperception.

With impairments noted in two forms of perception, testing for tactile perception was undertaken. Numbers were drawn on her fingerpads. She was unable to recognize them. Then the figures were drawn quite large on the palms of her hand. On the right side, she missed all of the numbers but gave the Gestaltian equivalents, that is, she identified 3 as 8, 6 as 2, 4 as 9. On the left side, she was somewhat better, but still interpreted half of the numbers incorrectly.

All three forms of perception were bad. On testing for motor function, it was discovered that it was impossible for her to perform separate motion on the two sides of her body at the same time. This was true whether the motions were the same or different. In tandem walking, she left spaces between her feet. At this point we moved her right foot backwards to show her that we wanted her heel and toe together. From this point on, she would put the right foot in front of her left one and then move it backwards to touch the left one. She would then put her left foot in the wrong position, but would not correct this. She obviously had problems with motor patterns.

This was a child with all forms of perceptual and motor dysfunction. Keeping her in a regular classroom would be a form of cruelty. This child needed help and lots of it, but she could be a productive person if given that help. One need look no further for evidence of her cleverness than the fact she had convinced her mother that she was an expert reader. The mother insisted her daughter read books to her. Upon questioning, the mother admitted the child sometimes substituted words that weren't in the book, and on a few occasions had read the book when it was upside down. She had even read four pages ahead of where she was looking. Obviously, the child had memorized the stories which her mother had first read to her.

In September of 1966, she returned to the same school setting which had resulted in two previous failures. There was no special facility available!

We would like to conclude this appeal for acceptance of neurological reading disorders by applying one question to these three cases: Does it seem that a "diagnosis does not have to be made," that a "few simple exercises . . . will quickly solve the problem"?

16.

Dyslexics Can Be Taught

Thus far a problem has been exposed that children are failing to learn to read because of unrecognized neurological disorders. It is a serious problem, not only because so many youngsters fail in this first task of education, but also because each case tends to be an individual one. These disabled readers cannot be categorized. Grouping them for instructional purposes will not be easy.

We have no solution to this problem. Nor do we believe there is *a* solution. There will have to be many solutions because of the variety of the disorders.

We believe physicians and psychologists can help in the search for solutions, but the main burden must lie with educators. Our nation's teachers are thoroughgoing experts in instruction. Many times in the past they have found ways to cope with very difficult educational problems, overcrowding, lack of qualified teachers, insufficient funds. They have learned to teach the deaf, the blind, the physically handicapped, the mentally retarded. When America was made aware of the need for more technically and scientifically trained personnel, schools regeared to emphasize these subjects. The illustration of the enterprise and dedication of teachers in the cause of improved education could go on to great length, but the point is we believe that teachers will be more than a match for the neurological problems we have endeavored to present here.

Solutions are possible. The McGlannan School in Miami, Florida, has reported excellent results in its efforts to teach dyslexics. It enrolls 65 youngsters with neurologic reading disorders and teaches them with a staff of 20. In its second year of operation, it has begun to develop pedagological approaches which permit children to be taught "individually" in small groups. Special emphasis is placed on multiple perceptual learning, simultaneously emphasizing visual, auditory and tactile *entrées* into language comprehension. The McGlannan School is certainly showing that solutions are possible.

In our practice, although the nature of a neurologist's clinical work regrettably does not often permit opportunity to follow a patient for many years, we have seen some problems solved.

Case No. 30. K.D. was a boy who had failed the second grade, principally because he was a behavior problem. He was withdrawn and antisocial, very quiet and unwilling to participate in class activities. His reading and spelling were unsatisfactory, but his arithmetic was above average.

He had excellent, concerned parents who took him to a speech and hearing clinic when he was in kindergarten. The history taken at the clinic showed that he was rather slow in maturation. He had sat at nine months and walked with help at 15 months, but did not walk unaided until his eighteenth month. He remained in the playpen until he was nearly two years old. Toilet training did not occur until he was three years old. His speech development was extremely slow. In kindergarten he did not yet speak in sentences. The clinicians observed: "In discussing the situation with the mother, one has the impression that the child has actually received very little speech and language stimulation directed to him. His demands have been so little that they have not paid much attention to him, and therefore it would seem wise to have every concerted effort made at this time toward speech and language stimulation from the family before we have further evaluation and/or speech therapy in the program. Mother was counseled at length on ways of doing simple speech and language stimulation for this youngster. What little we did, he appeared to enjoy and was interested in it." (We questioned the parental origin of his problem.)

The parents began working with the child. At the same time, the child was placed in a special educational setting which removed him from the frustration of the regular classroom. In hindsight, this was an excellent program. The root of the boy's reading difficulty appeared to be speech.

This young man was seen as a patient when he was ten and a half. His speech, still far from perfect, sounded like that of a person who had formerly had auditory imperception, which had improved, leaving him with a dysarthria, a speech defect. He was right-handed, but his left thumbnail was wider. Repetitive motion was done fairly well on the right, but poorly on the left. He had a moderate amount of mirror motion. He found it impossible to do independent motion, but his tandem walking was satisfactory. He was placed on medication.

In the months that followed, the program of speech emphasis was continued, along with regular remedial-reading instruction. When he was seen at eleven and a half, marked improvement had resulted. His motor difficulties had improved to the point of being almost normal, indicating that they had been maturational in nature. His speech was good, although on occasion he still had to search for a syllable or two. His Bender-Gestalt drawing showed normal visual perception. It was recommended to the school system that he be returned to a regular classroom at the fourth-grade level, only about a year behind in his schooling. This was done and remedial-reading instruction was continued, providing this boy with an excellent prognosis for the future.

This, then, was a patient who received help when he was young enough, thanks to his parents, and was given time in which the transient neurological disorders could improve. Deep emotional problems were avoided. It would be a mistake to assume such a program would work with all youngsters. Not all disorders are transient and the perceptual difficulties of others are so severe that much more intensive instruction is needed. But this case does indicate one possible solution to some problems.

Another solution is suggested by the following case:

Case No. 31. T.W. was a ten-year-old with a mild dysgraphia. He could read normally but writing was a major chore. He wrote quite slowly and made many errors. He had mixed handedness, writing left-handed, throwing right-handed, eating left-handed. His tactile perception was quite disordered. He misinterpreted numbers traced on the fingerpads of both hands, giving the

Gestaltian equivalents: 3 for 8, 4 for 9, 2 for 6, etc. His stereognosis was good, however.

This patient was seen intermittently for several years, most recently at age eighteen. At that time he was asked to copy in cursive writing some material out of a textbook. His effort is shown in Illustration 47.

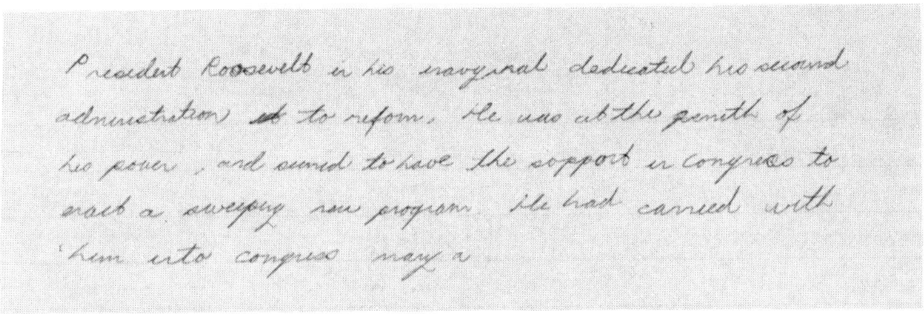

Illustration 47

What is significant about this is not the minor copying errors he made, but the fact it took him four minutes to perform this task! At age eighteen he still wrote agonizingly slowly. He was then asked to print the same passage. He was more accurate, but still required two minutes and 15 seconds to accomplish the task (Illustration 48).

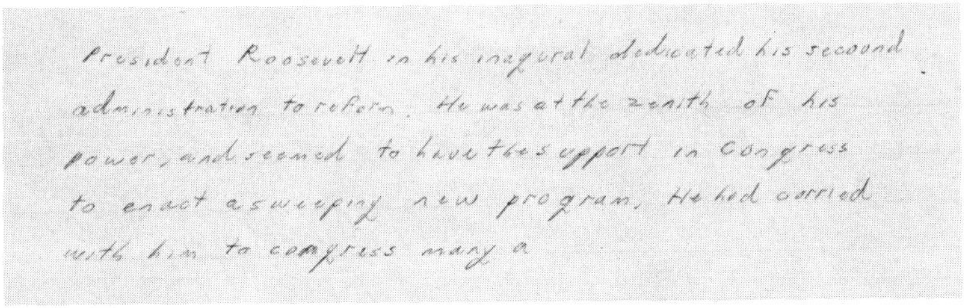

Illustration 48

Then the patient was asked to write some material to dictation. The result, in Illustration 49, is most unsatisfactory. He misspelled *prestige, pricked, court, reform, organize, industries* and other words and required two minutes and 45 seconds to do even this.

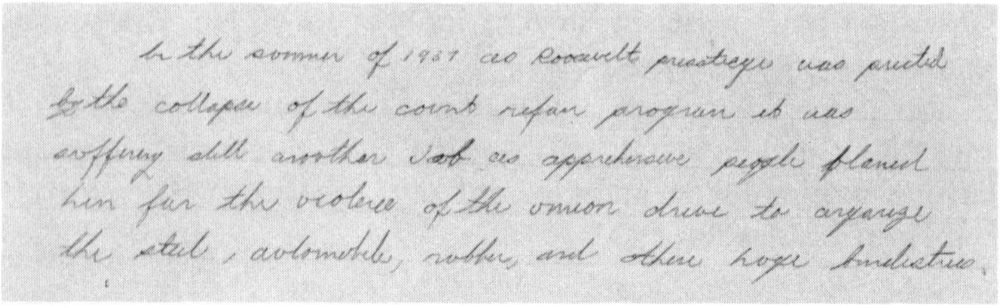

Illustration 49

This patient at age eighteen had a mild dysgraphia of a permanent nature. He knew he would always have it and accepted it with a shrug of the shoulders.

Was this fellow a failure in life? On the contrary, he had a great future ahead of him. He was due to graduate from high school in a few weeks with a ranking in the eightieth percentile of his class. He had been accepted by an excellent college, where he expected to major in political science. How could a child who wrote this badly graduate from high school? Quite simply: he didn't write. When he was first diagnosed at age ten, it was suggested that he learn to type. He went to summer school and learned. His parents bought him a portable typewriter, and he used it throughout school. He was also outfitted with a small portable tape recorder and, with the permission of school authorities, he used it instead of taking notes. When the teacher said something which ordinarily would require notes, he flicked on his tape recorder. All his themes and compositions were typewritten —to the joy of his teachers. Tests were administered to him either orally or individually so he could use his typewriter.

The point of this case is that this patient's neurological defect never was nor ever will be "cured." A way around the difficulty was found. It is not necessary in this age of typewriters and tape recorders for a person to be able to write. We believe that educators, when they put their minds to it, will be able to discover many other ways of avoiding problems that cannot be solved.

Case No. 32. E.C. was a boy of thirteen, a fifth-grade public-school student, referred by a pediatrician. Actually, he arrived for neurological examination by a more circuitous route. He had been arrested by the police for petty larceny from drugstores. Juvenile officers who questioned him felt there was something "wrong" with the boy and asked school authorities to investigate. E.C. was then tested by the school psychologist, his home environment was investigated by school social workers, and a physical examination was conducted. When all studies proved negative or inconclusive, a neurological examination was sought. It was most significant that this was not done until the thirteenth year of the boy's life and only then at the prodding of the police.

E.C.'s school and psychological records showed he had an IQ of 113, well above average, yet he had been a persistent school problem. His teacher reported, "This child doesn't like school. He doesn't pay attention in class. His mind wanders, and he looks out the window. I can't blame him for that, for he still reads at the first-grade level. Actually, he doesn't even know the alphabet. He is poor in arithmetic. He will fail again this year." School records showed he had failed the first, second, and third grades. When asked why he had passed the fourth, E.C. replied, "They had to paint the classroom." Thus, he was a teenage boy in the fifth grade who read at the first-grade level, even though, as his records showed, he had had four years of remedial-reading instruction. His school experience was one of repeated failure followed by what would appear to have been "social" promotions.

When seen as a patient, E.C. appeared to be healthy and of normal size and weight, good-looking and personable, although somewhat sullen. When asked what he would like to do more than anything else in the world, he replied, without hesitation, "I'd like to learn to read."

Neurological examination indicated a severe disorder of visual perception. On the Bender-Gestalt test, he performed approximately at the level of a seven-year-old. His tactile perception was also poor. There were no auditory or motor dysfunctions.

This boy was age thirteen when tested. Since impairments of perception often tend to improve with age, one can only imagine his perceptual difficulties when he was six years old and entering the first grade. Attempting to teach him to read by recognizing the shape of letters and words probably bordered on the impossible at that time, yet that was the method of instruction. Failure to learn to read was for him inevitable.

Because of the severity of this boy's problem and his high motivation to learn to read, a special effort was made. Following a conference with school officials, a remedial-reading instructor in his school volunteered to work with him during her lunch hour. Thus, he received 45 minutes a day, five days a week, of intensive instruction on a one-teacher-to-one-pupil basis. Fully cognizant of his perceptual difficulties, the teacher worked out a program to attempt to surmount them. She sought to improve his visual perception by pointing out the unique shapes of letters and patiently drilling him on letter recognition. More importantly, she emphasized phonics to make use of his normal auditory perception.

The methods used by this teacher, although experimental and tailored to the individual needs of this child, shed some light on ways other childen with visual imperception can be taught. She began by teaching her pupil to discriminate letter shapes. Together they discussed each letter as the boy wrote them on the blackboard, seeking ways in which he could discriminate each letter from its similar ones. After a great deal of drill—and much forgetfulness—the youngster began to be fairly consistent in recognizing and identifying the letters of the alphabet. His proficiency was further refined when the tutor used flash cards on which the individual letters were drawn. In time he was capable of instant recognition of each letter.

Then the teacher began simultaneous instruction in phonics and in sight recognition of words. The phonics instruction was quite conventional, with the child learning the sounds of the principal English phonemes. For this boy, who had no auditory imperception, this task was not particularly difficult once he had learned to identify the letters.

In the sight-recognition phase, the teacher concentrated on such short words as *the, off, to, two, too, not.* She used a flash-card technique, together with phonics. The boy would be shown the word, asked to recognize it and pronounce it phonically.

It took a full school year of one-to-one tutoring, 45 minutes a day, to enable this boy to read 300 words, but he had already overcome his biggest obstacles. He had the tools with which to expand his reading. In the second year, still using phonics and flash-card recognition, he progressed to increasingly longer and more complex words, then to phrases and sentences. At the end of the second year, he no longer had need for tutoring.

Many teachers doubtlessly would be able to improve on these techniques. In hindsight, we would say that perhaps more emphasis might have been placed on spelling patterns in the second year, yet the boy obviously became aware of these himself. The point we wish to make is that with the mild to moderate dyslexics, certainly, there is no particular mystique about teaching them. Once teachers are aware of the problems, once the children are recognized and diagnosed, once they are placed in the proper instructional setting, we have no doubt our teachers will be able to help them to learn to read.

Specific methods used in remedial reading have been discussed among therapists almost to the point of nausea. Many methods vary only slightly from one another, but it is the slight variation that is supposed to make a specific method more successful. As actually used, though, all theories fall into a few large groups, and all are derived from the basic ideas about the causes of reading disability.

Samuel T. Orton became interested in the dyslexic child in the 1920's and was a true pioneer in the study of learning problems in children. His concepts of *strephosymbolia* and *mixed dominance* became bywords in discussions of reading disabilities in the 1940's and 1950's. Anna Gillingham and Bessie Stillman, associated with him, devised a method now known as the Orton-Gillingham Approach. Originally designated the "alphabetic method," it has been modified through the years into a visual-auditory-kinesthetic method. This is not a fixed protocol, as can be seen from J. L. Orton's statement in 1966:

> Every remedial tutor must experiment to a certain extent with each individual pupil in the application of basic principles of retraining, such as those of the Orton-Gillingham Approach. Experience with many pupils will gradually lead to the teacher's own preferred procedures. These in turn will be passed on to others in training and will become the starting point for the development of individual batteries of effective techniques.[1]

The Orton-Gillingham Approach is basically a phonic one in which the association of phoneme to grapheme is taught by auditory, visual and kinesthetic (voice and writing) methods. Directionality is also stressed by the Orton school in the diagnosis and remediation of reading difficulties.

To this background, Grace Fernald added the tactile element, and as a result many VAKT (visual-auditory-kinesthetic-tactile) methods have arisen. The tactile element involves the feeling and manipulation of letters to learn their shape. The letters may be made of many substances—wood, plastic, sandpaper—or even traced in sandboxes. There are now an infinite number of VAKT protocols practiced by various remediationists.

The importance in reading disability of early development of visual discrimination seemed of great significance to Marian Frostig, a pioneer in the study of the development of children. The Frostig Test for Visual Discrimination[2] explores the function in five different modalities. On the basis of the test, a remedial method was constructed to correct difficulties in any or all of these five areas. This technique is still used extensively with children having demonstrable disorder of visual discrimination.

It is a pity that no one has worked out a system of identifying characteristics for all the letters of the alphabet, as suggested by Gibson's work (see pages 75 and 76). Such a system adapted for teaching would be a great aid to those whose problem is the visual discrimination of letters.

All of the above basic approaches have been modified, added to and mixed, to give an almost infinite variety. But these are concerned only with the recognition of letters and the association of the letters with sounds. Kephart thought that motor development was important and stressed body image, rhythm, directionality, coordination, fine muscle control, ocular control and so forth, in a testing device as well as in an extensive therapeutic system.[3] According to this concept, stressing the area of motor development positively influences reading ability through stimulating brain development. Although this technique is not generally applied as a whole, portions of it remain in frequent practice, as can be seen from the number of physical training programs still considered part of therapy in remediation centers.

Counter to the "phonic revolution," E. W. Dolch developed a remedial program based on a sight method. Because of its neglect of phonics this approach has fallen into disuse and is often thought of as regressive. Nevertheless the Dolch Word List (most common words given by age level) is a much used research instrument, and there are many children today with auditory problems who would profit from such a program.

As can be seen, none of these methods takes into account language disorders. We found it necessary to design a remediation program for children having language difficulties. We have attempted to teach these children to read by converting a mark on paper into a concept, eliminating the interval steps of sound and language. To do this, we have combined sight reading with rebus reading (in a rebus, a pictographic symbol represents a word or phoneme; for example, a picture of an eye is read as *I*).

The method consists of using two sets of cards; one set has the required words printed on them, and the other set has pictures illustrating these words. When the instructor holds up the card with the letters *c-a-t*, the student holds up the card with a picture of a cat. Nothing is said. Whether the student conceives of *c-a-t* as meaning "says meow," "catches mice" or "a cat" makes no difference. He can be taught to retrieve the concept appropriate to the alphabetic word even if he cannot retrieve the specific word.

The child taught by this system can "read" for comprehension very accurately and rapidly—in fact, often much more rapidly than the routinely taught reader—but he cannot read word for word orally. He cannot be called upon to read in class, but he can maintain his grade level, or perform above it, in comprehension. By intermediate school age he begins to associate words with their graphic images and, as natural development and well-directed therapy improve his language skills, he becomes a fluent silent reader with passable oral ability.

Some have objected to this method as a regressive return to silent reading. But, as Gibson has shown, with age and experience sight readers involuntarily learn a phonic system. By using this sight-rebus method, those with language-based dyslexia can become successful intermediate and secondary school students without distortion of self-image, and often more rapid readers eventually than their peers. (See page 48.)

We cannot say that any one particular method is better than any other. The choice of method should be related to the need of the child involved and, therefore, depends solely on the specificity of the diagnosis and the eclecticism of the therapist. In short, the best method for any particular child uses his abilities, avoids his disabilities and is successful.

17.

Some Thoughts about Solutions

AT SEVERAL POINTS in this book we have suggested that three academic disciplines are involved in reading instruction. The psychologist should study the normal reading process. The physician should pursue the causes of abnormal reading—and, this book notwithstanding, we emphasize *pursue*, for our knowledge of reading disorders is far from complete. The teacher should be primarily concerned with therapy and the development of techniques of teaching both normal and abnormal children to read.

Of these three disciplines, the educator and the psychologist have performed best through the years. Our progress in the teaching of reading is the result largely of their efforts. But even this leaves something to be desired, as Eleanor J. Gibson, the Cornell psychologist, has pointed out:[1]

> Educators and the public have exhibited a keen interest in the teaching of reading ever since free public education became a fact. Either because of or despite their interest, this most important subject has been remarkably susceptible to the influence of fads and fashions and curiously unaffected by disciplined experimental and theoretical psychology. The psychologists have traditionally pursued the study of verbal learning by means of experiments with nonsense syllables and the like—that is, materials carefully divested of useful information. And the educators, who found little in this work that seemed relevant to the classroom, have stayed with the classroom; when they performed experiments, the method was apt to be a gross comparison of classes privileged and unprivileged with respect to the latest fad. The result has been two cultures: the pure scientists in the laboratory

and the practical teachers ignorant of the progress that has been made in the theory of human learning and in methods of studying it. That this split was unfortunate was clear enough.

If the alliance between educators and psychologists has not always been fully productive, the physician has contributed even less. He gives physical examinations and treats physical ailments, but in the instruction of reading, he has remained a spectator. The doctor has considered himself no more an expert in reading instruction than any other member of the PTA.

Even neurologists, those medical specialists most concerned with brain function, have until recently contributed little that is useful to the classroom teacher. There have been neurological studies, to be sure, going back to Déjerine in the nineteenth century, but the studies have been on adults who have lost the ability to read and on children with abnormal neurological function. Studying persons who have suffered a stroke or other injury and thus lost the ability to read is useful to people so afflicted, but it does not contribute much to the study of the child who has never learned to read. Similarly, the neurological studies of retarded or so-called "brain-damaged" children have produced admirable results in teaching these youngsters to read, but unfortunately this is not very helpful in understanding the teaching of reading to the normal child.

Learning to read is a different process than reacquiring an ability to read which has been lost. Adults who have lost the ability can use, in relearning, their previously learned abilities which were not impaired, such as writing or an extensive vocabulary. At the very least the adult who is relearning to read knows what the reading process is, a fact which the first-grade child must discover.

Others have commented on the fallacy of misapplying adult studies to the normal child. Dr. M. D. Vernon, a leading psychologist, has written,[2]

> When adults study and assess children's ability to read, they are apt to consider this ability as a single homogeneous entity. This is not unnatural, for in educated adults reading has become a firmly established habitual activity which they perform with great ease and speed. Consequently they are unaware of the various processes which they themselves must carry out in reading. And they do not recognize that children who are in the early stages of read-

ing may utilize procedures which are quite different from those employed by adults. In such children, reading is not a well-organized system of habits. A child must go laboriously through a number of interrelated activities before he can fully understand the meaning of printed words and sentences. He may stumble or break down at any stage in the proceedings. Such a failure may interfere badly with the whole process of reading, and the child will appear to be a backward reader or even an illiterate.

It seems to us that solutions to the reading problem in this country require, as a first step, the united and coordinated action of psychologists, educators and physicians. The controversy, jealousy and often downright bickering which have characterized much of the effort to solve the reading problem are both immature and regrettable. Entirely too much educational thought has been negative.

There is a most unfortunate tendency on the part of some educators—a differentiation from teachers is important here—to square off into camps. These various educational cliques are customarily able to unite, however, to reject and repel any attempts by "outsiders," such as psychologists, physicians, parents and public officials, to "interfere" with education.

TEACHER ATTITUDES

The classroom teacher plays a crucial role in any educational program for dyslexics. Above all, teachers need to accept the existence of these disorders. If teachers believe neurological reading disorders are in the category of snake-oil remedies and witchcraft, then no solution is possible. If the facts of these disorders are accepted, then the teachers, psychologists and remedial-reading clinicians must learn when to suspect that a child may have a neurological disorder and arrange for a detailed study of the child.

The teacher's responsibility for recognizing the dyslexic child is clear-cut. Only in the very severe and unusual cases will the child's neurological problems reveal themselves before the child starts to school. Parents cannot be expected to detect the perceptual impairments which characterize dyslexia. Only the teacher hears the child read and observes his struggles to distinguish letters and to write them. She alone is able to compare the dyslexic child's performance with that of the normal child. As we have pointed out, the severe problems will show up quite early in the first grade. The moderate disability may be demonstrated later in the first grade. Some of the mild dyslexics may not be recognized until the second or third grade.

The child who is a suspected dyslexic must receive a careful, thorough diagnosis which pinpoints the nature and extent of his perceptual (and other) disorders so that a program of instruction can be constructed for him. We realize this is a rather pat statement. An examination by a neurologist is not always practical. Neurology is not one of the popular medical specialties, and most neurologists are congregated in large cities. There are sections of the country where there is no properly trained neurologist within hundreds of miles. And many neurologists have not been interested in dyslexia. The gross neurological maladies, such as muscular dystrophy and multiple sclerosis, have had more appeal. Complex cases of dyslexia will probably always require a neurological consultation, but in practice many pediatricians and some psychiatrists have been making these diagnoses. The sheer volume of the reading problem and the concern of parents has forced non-neurologically trained physicians to "bone up" on neurology in order to help their patients. There is no particular medical mystique about diagnosing dyslexia. A pediatrician who makes a special study of it can easily become a diagnostician. It would be more than helpful, however, if the curriculum of medical schools was altered to include material about dyslexia in pediatric training.

After diagnosis is made, the teacher must have empathy for the child. She must accept his limitations and, while working to improve them, view them with the same attitude she would have to the fact he had blue eyes, or was left-handed, color blind, tone deaf, or blond-haired.

A portion of the mild dyslexics can remain in the regular classroom if some specific actions are taken—or not taken. We believe it is important that he not be called upon regularly to reveal his disability. What is gained by having him read orally before the class? He needs to read orally, to be sure, but does he have to do it before his peers, amid snickering and ridicule? How much better if he reads more privately and in an atmosphere of understanding and acceptance. If he has dysgraphia, is it absolutely necessary that he hand in his papers and be graded on a par with the normal youngsters in his class? Or, can some allowance be made for his misspelling, his intent, his information? And why can't he be tested orally?

All of this comes under the category of teacher attitude. If a teacher has a class containing a couple of mildly dyslexic, dysgraphic youngsters, she has a responsibility to help the children and to protect them from emotional problems. The other pupils in the class will reflect the teacher's attitude. If she believes that the child's disorder is socially acceptable, that he is intelligent, and that the ability to read and write is not a mark of intelligence, that he can contribute to the class and to society despite his limitation, that he is, in short, a fine person, then the other members of the class will share her attitude—and the dyslexic child will, too.

The teacher of the mildly dyslexic child in a regular classroom has a responsibility to see that this child receives remedial reading. In our experience too many teachers look upon the poor reader as a mark of their personal failure. If they don't teach a child to read well, it is their fault and they are poor teachers. This is nonsense. Giving the dyslexic child the individual attention he needs is beyond possibility for the teacher with 25, 30 or more students in a class. If she does, she is neglecting the other students. The teacher should send the mildly dyslexic child to remedial-reading classes, and she ought to consider it a mark of her astuteness that she sends as many children as need be to such classes. It indicates she is aware of the problems of the children in her charge.

REMEDIAL READING

The remedial-reading instruction, as we have emphasized, must be tailored to fit the unique needs of each individual dyslexic. Ideally, each child ought to have an hour a day of tutoring on a one-teacher-to-one-pupil basis. But that goal is utopian. Individual tutoring sessions cost ten to fifteen dollars an hour. With three to four million youngsters in need of this instruction, an expenditure of 150 million dollars a week would be required. It might be argued that such a vast expenditure is worth it to teach these children, but, pragmatically, such funds are never going to be available.

The alternative is for remedial-reading instructors to find a way to teach small groups of these youngsters. Three to six children with similar disorders (visual imperception, for example) could perhaps be drilled as a unit on the distinguishing characteristics of letters. If the members of the unit all had unimpaired auditory perception, they could receive together the training in phonics which is so essential for them. If they had no tactile difficulties, they could write letters in sand, make them with clay or pipe cleaners, work with block letters and the other kinesthetic means.

This group would have to be carefully selected following diagnosis, but in a school system of moderate size, groups could be formulated consisting of dyslexics with visual imperception alone, auditory imperception alone, visual imperception with tactile difficulties, visual and tactile with motor disorders, etc. It is reasonable to assume that a small group of youngsters with similar problems of more or less equal severity could be taught together.

The question of severity of the disability is vital to any therapeutic program. Any remedial reading, even the worst in the world, will help the mildly dyslexic child. Unfortunately, a substantial portion of schools either have no remedial programs or are grossly understaffed. We recently wrote to the principal of a suburban school suggesting that a patient receive remedial reading. We received the following reply:

> Since entering our school as a second-grade repeater, this boy was immediately diagnosed as a severe reading problem. He was classified as a "non-reader" who needed intensive instruction. He was placed on the list for the county reading clinic, but was not selected to attend. [As a matter of fact, the patient was on the list for two years.] To make a long story short, this patient has been diagnosed as having average intelligence, does have the ability to learn, but has never been presented with the proper intensive instruction he needs. Most of this can be attributed to the fact that this school is one of the few in the county without a remedial- or corrective-reading teacher. Last month I requested such a teacher for next year's program. Any words you can properly place to help insure us of this teacher would be greatly ap-

preciated. Until we can offer this boy the program he needs, I'm afraid that his prognosis will be no better than his past achievements.

The magnitude of the reading problem in this country cries aloud for a great increase in appropriations for remedial-reading classes. Even where such programs exist and where a child is enrolled, the procedure is not properly geared to help the Waysiders. The classes are too big, for one thing. More than six youngsters to a group is self-defeating. Then, there is often a hopeless mishmash of reading problems in the same class. This is not universally true, but it is true entirely too often. Even the worst remedial reading will help the mildly dyslexic child, but many classes would benefit from simple organization.

SPECIAL CLASSES

The mild dyslexic can usually remain in the regular classroom if (1) he is recognized early; (2) he has an understanding teacher; and (3) he receives regular, hopefully daily, remedial reading in a special class setting.

The moderate-to-severe dyslexic poses a more difficult problem. He needs a great deal of very precise, individualized reading instruction for several years. He cannot possibly remain in a regular classroom.

The educational problem of the moderate-to-severe dyslexic is twofold. First, he must learn to read as well as he is able, obviously in remedial-reading classes. Second, he must receive information. The ultimate tragedy of these youngsters is that their reading problem denies them information. Our whole educational process after the third grade is geared to learning by reading. If the child cannot read at grade level, he is denied history, geography, science, government, all the facts and concepts a normal child receives. His intellectual capacity diminishes and his IQ scores tail off, sometimes markedly.

An important task of the public-school system, in the United States certainly, is to teach a child to read. But the schools' larger duty is to teach the information which helps create an enlightened, educated person. In a regular classroom, the moderate-to-severe dyslexic child is denied this information. He is intelligent. He can learn in ways other than by reading: orally by being read to or in lectures by the teacher; movies and film strips; television; discussion groups among the students; visiting lecturers; field trips. Once they put their minds to it, teachers could work out many clever ways to teach information other than by reading. In the elementary grades, the dyslexic child could learn as much information by oral means as the normal child does by reading.

Such a program of instruction would involve special oral classes, consisting of 25 or 30 moderate-to-severe dyslexics. For a portion of the day they would receive remedial reading and during the remainder they would learn information. This would be a much different class than regular ones. Movies, television, displays and other visual aids would be important paraphernalia, along with auditory aids such as tape recorders, phonographs, radios, loudspeaker systems. As the situation warranted, the individual students might carry small tape recorders.

A school system of moderate-to-large size would certainly have enough dyslexic children to warrant setting up such classes, just as there are classes for the retarded, physically handicapped, blind and deaf. In rural areas, such classes might have to be established on a county or other centralized basis. But we see such classes as the only realistic solution to the informational problems of the severe dyslexic.

The curriculum and other mechanics of setting up and operating such special classes is beyond the skein of our experience. Educators, with their expertise and experience, could do this with relative ease. But we might suggest that consideration be given to this format: for the severely dyslexic children, eliminate all reading instruction for the first five years. Concentrate entirely on teaching these children information by means that do not require reading. Limit reading to those handful of words essential to their safety, such as *stop, fire, danger, poison,* etc. They will want to know their name, address and telephone number. Then, when these children are ten or twelve, begin intensive reading instruction. At this age, when the children are more neurologically mature, many of the perceptual and other disorders which plagued them as six-year-olds will have improved or disappeared. At this age they can be taught to read, at least as well as they are ever going to, with far, far greater speed and much less effort, expense and exasperation. We realize the novelty of such a suggestion. We may have neglected factors which make it impractical. But we offer it for consideration.

ESTABLISHING A PROGRAM FOR DYSLEXICS

Miss Dorothy G. Sleep, principal of the Kings Highway Elementary School in Westport, Connecticut, who read the manuscript of this book, asked how a school system could undertake to establish a program to aid dyslexics.

The first step, it seems to us, is for the school system to hold a workshop or seminar on dyslexia for elementary teachers, remedial-reading teachers, psychologists, supervisors and others involved in the school reading program. By lectures, papers and other suitable means, the classroom teacher should learn how to detect the various forms of dyslexia. This is the crucial step. We must start identifying the children with neurological reading disorders.

Second, we suggest that a committee be established consisting of a psychologist, the school reading therapist, a physician acquainted with dyslexia, and an educational administrator familiar with the problems of school finances, classroom availability, teacher assignments and the other logistics of school operation. This committee should then arrange for each suspected dyslexic child to be examined by the reading therapist, the psychologist and the physician to develop a precise diagnosis of the nature of the child's reading disorder. Together with the educational "logician," they should endeavor to work out the best remedial program presently available in the school system.

There is immediacy, even urgency, to these suggestions. These steps can and should be taken right now. The results will be only stopgap, but they will be a move in the right direction.

We must also proceed toward long-range solutions. We need to know, for example, how to teach a child to read. If the findings of the Cornell University study are correct, many of our present methods of reading instruction are wasteful and even self-defeating. The studies begun at Cornell need to be expanded and pursued. Experimental classes need to be established to test these various theories and discover the best methodology for teaching reading to normal children. Experimental classes need to be created for various types of dyslexic children. How can these children be grouped? What is the best age to begin instruction? How much instruction is feasible at one time? Can visual, auditory and tactile perception be improved by instruction? What type of remedial program is most effective for the various disorders? How can the dyslexics receive information while learning to read? Would some form of Initial Perceptual Alphabet be practical? Is the basal-reader, language-experience or individual-learning (or some other) method of instruction the best? What sort of readers should the dyslexics have?

The questions proliferate and there are no answers. This is true in the realm of medicine as fully as in psychology and education: How may diagnostic techniques be improved? What is the nature of brain maturation? Is there some way· maturation can be altered? Is medical treatment for perceptual problems possible? Neurologists are required to answer "We don't know" far too often, for we are only on the threshold of understanding brain function.

It would be a shame if this vast educational, psychological and medical research program grew like Topsy. It will be far more efficacious and inexpensive if it has leadership. It needs to be coordinated by a large university or educational association and financed by government and foundations. With proper coordination, a teacher in Tuscaloosa or Boise could undertake experimental work, perhaps as part of her master's or doctorate work, which was integrated with, rather than duplicative of, an experiment in Buffalo or Sacramento. Such a plan may be hopelessly utopian, but then so was the whole scheme of free public education.

PARENTAL ATTITUDES

Mothers and fathers have a role in any educational program for the dyslexic child. It is said the dyslexic child (and all children) needs the Three A's—Acceptance, Approval, Affection. Parents need to accept and understand the child's disorder, just as they would if he had a gross malady such as blindness or congenital heart disease. It's a case of "That's the way he is, love him." The pressure for excellence must be removed. He should not be badgered, ridiculed, compared to others, threatened or punished. Nor should parents be permissive. He should not be babied, coddled or excused. The parents—and the child—should have a realistic appraisal of his limitation and expected performance. The child should be asked to do as well as he is able—but not better than that. He should understand that because of his limitation he will have to work harder to achieve less results than his nondyslexic buddies. That is the way the ball of life has bounced. If a child has useless legs and must walk on crutches, good parents know that, as difficult as it may be for them, they should not pick up the child when he falls. He must struggle to his feet himself, for in life there will not always be someone to assist him. If a child is blind, he must learn to walk with a cane or other means, for he cannot go through life hanging on the arm of a companion. So it is with the dyslexic child. He must learn to do as well as he can and then adjust his life to his limitations.

Believe it or not, it is not necessary to be an expert reader in this life. One can learn orally. One can tape-record what others say or hire someone to read to him and a secretary to take dictation. Many dyslexics have trained their memories to high levels of efficiency. Poor readers can be expert mechanics, technicians, businessmen, artists, athletes, physicians, some types of engineer, salesmen, photographers, to name a few. Dyslexia is a handicap to be surmounted, and surmounting a handicap builds character. Consider Helen Keller or Franklin Delano Roosevelt and thousands more.

The task of the parents is to help the child make best use of his ability, however limited. If dyslexia is suspected, have him diagnosed. If the school lacks a suitable program, parents can help get one started or perhaps arrange for some tutoring. In our opinion, even if they feel qualified, parents should not attempt the tutoring themselves. Like a physician treating his own child, the parents are too emotionally involved with the dyslexic to teach him. The parents' role is that of support, offering acceptance, approval and affection that will enable the child to surmount his handicap.

We hope in conclusion that, despite its limitations, this book will light some spark, that as a nation we can begin to reach out our hands to those neurologically impaired children who stand by the wayside of education.

Bibliographical Notes

CHAPTER 1

1. Fries, Charles C. *Linguistics and Reading.* New York: Holt, Rinehart and Winston, 1962, p. 1.
2. Holt, John. *How Children Fail.* New York: Dell, 1964, p. 9.

CHAPTER 2

1. Westman, Jack C., Arthur, Bettie, and Scheidler, Edward P. "Reading Retardation: An Overview," *Am. J. Dis. Child.*, 109 (1965), 359–369.
2. The high estimate of 75 percent is from Walcutt, Charles C., "The Reading Problem in America," in *Tomorrow's Illiterates, The State of Reading Today,* Charles C. Walcutt, editor (Boston: Little, Brown, 1961), p. 11. The low limit of 10 percent is by Cronin, Sister Eileen Marie, "Reading Disorders and Remediation," in *Reading Disorders, A Multidisciplinary Symposium,* Richard M. Flower, Helen F. Gofman and Lucie I. Lawson, editors (Philadelphia: F. A. Davis, 1965), p. 104. Between the two extremes many estimates may be found. The two most recent are: Walton, George H., "Why Half Our Draftees Flunk," *This Week Magazine* (New York: United Newspapers Magazine, March 13, 1966), p. 2 (25 percent); and Ellingson, Careth, and Cass, James, "New Hope for Non-Readers," *Saturday Review of Literature* (April 16, 1966), p. 82 (20 percent). As for specific figures on dyslexia, an estimate of 10 to 15 percent has been

given by: O'Sullivan, Mary Ann, and Pryles, Victor A., "Reading Disability in Children," *J. Pediat.*, 60(1962):369–375; and Hawke, William A., "Specific Reading Disabilities," *Pediat. Clinics N. Amer.*, May 1958, 513–522.

3. That reading difficulty plays a major role in the production of the school dropout and the delinquent is well documented in *The School Dropout*, Daniel Schreiber, editor (Washington: National Education Association, 1964), particularly the article by Warren G. Findley entitled "Language Development and Dropouts." Also: Roman, Melvin, *Reaching Delinquents Through Reading*. Springfield, Illinois: Charles C Thomas, 1957.

4. Woodring, Paul, in Cronin, *op. cit.*, p. 104. Hechinger, Fred M., "College Pressures," *The New York Times*, Sunday, April 25, 1965.

5. Fries, Charles C., *op. cit.*, pp. 4–5.

6. Mann, Horace, as quoted by Walcutt, Charles C., *op. cit.*, p. 27.

7. Fries, Charles C., *op. cit.*, p. 5.

8. Gray, W. S., as quoted by Fries, Charles C., *op. cit.*, p. 3.

9. Downing, John. *The Initial Teaching Alphabet*. London: Cassell and Co., 3rd edition, 1964.

10. Harris, Albert J. *How to Increase Reading Ability: A Guide to Developmental and Remedial Methods*. New York: Longmans, Green, 1956.

11. Walcutt, Charles C., *op. cit.*, p. 16.

12. Goldberg, Herman K. National Conference on Dyslexia, Philadelphia, November, 1966.

13. Critchley, Macdonald. *Developmental Dyslexia*. Springfield, Illinois: Charles C. Thomas, 1964, p. 45.

14. Gray, William S., Kibbe, Delia, Lucas, Laura, and Miller, Lawrence W., as quoted by Robinson, Helen M. *Why Pupils Fail in Reading*. Chicago: University of Chicago Press, 1946, p. 59.

15. Olson, Willard C. "Reading as a Function of the Total Growth of the Child," in *Reading and Pupil Development*, William S. Gray, editor. (Supplemental Educational Monographs No. 51) Chicago: University of Chicago Press, 1940, pp. 233–237.

16. Durrell, Donald D. *Improvement of Basic Reading Abilities*. New York: World Book, 1940.

CHAPTER 3

1. Burton, William H. *Reading in Child Development*. New York: Bobbs-Merrill, 1956, p. 19.
2. McKee, Paul. *The Teaching of Reading in the Elementary School*. Boston: Houghton Mifflin, 1948.
3. Hester, Kathleen B. *Teaching Every Child to Read*. New York: Harper & Row, 2nd edition, 1964, p. 2.
4. Carey, Helen B. "The Bright Underachiever in Reading. Causes of Underachievement," in *The Underachiever in Reading*. H. Alan Robinson, editor. Chicago: University of Chicago Press, 1962, p. 75.

CHAPTER 4

1. Dietrich, Coralie. "Changes in Reading Achievement, Perceptual Motor Ability, and Behavior Adjustment as a Function of Perceptual Motor Training and Individualized Remedial Reading Instruction," February, 1972. Project No. O–E–104, U.S. Office of Education.
2. Ausubel, David P. *The Psychology of Meaningful Verbal Learning*. New York: Grune & Stratton, 1963, p. 31.
3. McCarthy, Dorothea. "Language Development in Children," in *Manual of Child Psychology*, Leonard Carmichael, editor. New York: John Wiley and Sons, 1946, p. 482.
4. *Ibid.*, p. 506.
5. Bloomfield, Leonard. "Linguistics and Reading," in *Elementary Engl. Rev.* 19:125–130, 183–186, 1942.

CHAPTER 5

1. The Cornell University study, *A Basic Research Program on Reading*, consists of 22 separate papers which are not sequentially numbered, so that page references would be of little significance. Because copies of the full report are difficult to obtain, additional references will be listed for each paper, if published elsewhere. The papers discussed in this chapter are:

Gibson, Eleanor J., Gibson, James J., Pick, Anne D., and Osser, Harry. "A Developmental Study of the Discrimination of Letter-Like Forms" (also published in *J. Comp. Physiol. Psychol.*, 55:897–905, 1962).

Gibson, Eleanor J., Osser, Harry, Schiff, William, and Smith, Jesse. "An Analysis of Critical Features of Letters, Tested by a Confusion Matrix."

Pick, Anne D. "Improvement in Visual Discrimination of Letter-Like Forms" (also published in *J. Exp. Psychol.*, 69:331, 1965).

Gibson, James J., and Osser, Harry. "A Possible Effect of Learning to Write on Learning to Read."

Edelman, Gabrielle. "The Use of Cues in Word Recognition."

2. Gibson, Eleanor J. "Learning to Read," in *Science,* 148 (May 21, 1965), 1066–1072.

3. Mowbray, R. M., and Rodger, T. Ferguson. *Psychology in Relation to Medicine.* Edinburgh: E. and S. Livingstone, 1963, p. 208.

4. *Stedman's Medical Dictionary.* London: Bailliere, Tindall & Cox, 1961.

5. Hebb, D. O. *The Organization of Behavior.* London: John Wiley and Sons, 1949, pp. 31–33.

6. *Ibid.*, p. 36.

7. Brown, Roger. "A Dispute About Reading," in *Human Learning in the School,* John P. DeCecco, ed. New York: Holt, Rinehart and Winston, 1964, p. 348. (Reprinted from Brown, Roger: *Words and Things.* Glencoe, Illinois: The Free Press, 1959, p. 73.)

8. Gibson, Eleanor J., *op. cit.*, p. 1068.

9. Fernald, Grace. *Remedial Techniques in Basic School Subjects.* London: McGraw-Hill, 1943.

CHAPTER 6

1. Gibson, Eleanor J., *op. cit.*, p. 1069.

2. The individual papers from *A Basic Research Program on Reading* discussed in this chapter are:

Bishop, Carol. "Transfer of Word and Letter Training in Reading" (also published in *J. Verbal Learning Verbal Behav.*, 3:215, 1964).

Levin, Harry and Watson, John. "The Learning of Variable Grapheme-to-Phoneme Correspondences."

Levin, Harry and Watson, John. "The Learning of Variable Grapheme-to-Phoneme Correspondences: Variations in the Initial Consonant Position."

Levin, Harry, Baum, Esther, and Bostwick, Susan. "The Learning of Variable Grapheme-to-Phoneme Correspondences: Comparison of English and Spanish Speakers."

Gibson, Eleanor J., Pick, Anne D., Osser, Harry, and Hammond, Marcia. "The Role of Grapheme-Phoneme Correspondence in the Perception of Words" (also published in *Am. J. Psychol.*, 75:554, 1962).

Gibson, Eleanor J., Osser, Harry, and Pick, Anne D., "A Study of the Development of Grapheme-Phoneme Correspondences" (also published in *J. Verbal Learning Verbal Behav.*, 2:142, 1963).

Gibson, Eleanor J., Bishop, Carol H., Schiff, William, and Smith, Jesse. "A Comparison of Meaningfulness and Pronounceability as Grouping Principles in the Perception and Retention of Verbal Material" (also published in *J. Exp. Psychol.*, 67:173, 1964).

3. Bloomfield, Leonard, *op. cit.*

4. Brown, Roger, *op. cit.*, p. 349 (p. 75).

5. Gibson, Eleanor J., *op. cit.*, p. 1071.

6. *Ibid.*

CHAPTER 7

1. Critchley, Macdonald. *Developmental Dyslexia, op. cit.*, p. 77.

2. Bredsdorff, E., as quoted by Critchley, M., *ibid.*, p. 72.

3. Hermann, Knud. *Reading Disability. A Medical Study of Word-Blindness and Related Handicaps*. Translated by P. G. Aungle. Springfield, Illinois: Charles C. Thomas, 1959, p. 150.

4. Critchley, Macdonald. *The Parietal Lobes*. London: E. Arnold, 1953, p. 359.

5. Ingram, T. T. S. "Pediatric Aspects of Specific Developmental Dysphasia, Dyslexia and Dysgraphia," *Cerebral Palsy Bull.*, 2:254–277, 1960.

6. Orton, S. T. *Reading, Writing and Speech Problems in Children*. New York: W. W. Norton, 1937, p. 142.

7. Critchley, Macdonald. *Developmental Dyslexia, op. cit.,* p. 76.

8. Halgren, B. "Specific Dyslexia (Congenital Word-Blindness): Clinical and Genetic Study," *Acta Psychiat. Neurol.,* suppl. 65:1–287, 1950.

9. Vernon, M. D. *Backwardness in Reading.* Cambridge: Cambridge University Press, 1957.

10. Drew, A. I. "A Neurologic Appraisal of Familial Congenital Word-Blindness," *Brain,* 79:440–460, 1956.

11. Hermann, Knud, *op. cit.,* p. 44.

12. Critchley, Macdonald, *Developmental Dyslexia, op. cit.*

13. Denhoff, Eric. "Bridges to Burn and to Build," *Develop. Med. and Child Neurol.,* 7:3–8 1965.

14. *Time Magazine.* "Education: Reading, Some Johnnies Just Can't," May 13, 1966.

15. Orton, S. T., *op. cit.,* p. 200.

16. Penfield, Wilder, and Robertson, J. S. M. "Growth Asymmetry Due to Cerebral Lesions of the Postcentral Cortex," *Arch. Neurol. and Psychiat.,* 50:405–430, 1943. For the introduction to this concept of nail size in relation to handedness and cerebral function, the author is indebted to Dr. Douglas N. Buchanan.

17. Drew, S. I., *op. cit.,* p. 457.

18. Brain, R., as quoted by Whitsell, Leon J. "Neurologic Aspects of Reading Disorders," in *Reading Disorders, op. cit.,* p. 49.

19. Zangwill, O. L. "Dyslexia in Relation to Cerebral Dominance," in *Reading Disability,* J. Money, editor. Baltimore: Johns Hopkins Press, 1962, p. 112.

CHAPTER 8

1. Bender, Lauretta. *A Visual Motor Gestalt Test and Its Clinical Use.* New York: American Orthopsychiatric Association, 1938.

2. Glaser, Kurt, and Clemmens, Raymond L. "School Failure," *Pediatrics,* 35:128–141, 1965.

CHAPTER 9

1. Hermann, Knud, *op. cit.,* p. 45.

CHAPTER 10

1. The term *dysgraphia* is a difficult one. When defined as "inability to write, caused by a cerebral lesion" (*Random House Dictionary of the English Language*. New York: Random House, 1966, p. 446), the concept is incomplete. When we use *dysgraphia* we refer to an abnormal disability in spelling, both verbal and written, existing in the presence of normal intelligence, motor function, speech and possibly reading ability, which is resistant to all teaching, and due to a dysfunction of the cerebral cortex. In the presence of normal visual perception, the dysgraphic individual can copy accurately. This term should not be used to describe a purely motor disability as illustrated in Illustration 44 in Chapter 12.

CHAPTER 11

1. Hermann, Knud, *op. cit.*, p. 134.
2. *Ibid.*, pp. 106–147.
3. Critchley, Macdonald. *The Parietal Lobes, op. cit.*, Chapter VII.

CHAPTER 12

1. The term *apraxia* is used here in a liberal or perhaps English or Jacksonian way rather than in the sense that Liepmann and the German neurologists used it. We are trying to indicate a purely ideomotor disorder rather than a language or aphasic one. Our patients cannot perform a patterned action whether the instruction is by command or demonstration. Thus "an inability to perform purposeful movements, but not accompanied by a loss of sensory function or paralysis" (*Random House Dictionary of the English Language, op. cit.*, p. 74), or "a disorder of voluntary movement consisting in a more or less complete incapacity to execute purposeful movements, notwithstanding the preservation of muscular power, sensibility and coordination in general" (*Stedman's Medical Dictionary, op. cit.*).
2. Luria, A. R. "Two Kinds of Motor Perseveration in Massive Injury to the Frontal Lobes," *Brain*, 88:1, 1965.

CHAPTER 13

1. Benton, Arthur L. "Developmental Aphasia and Brain Damage," *Cortex*, 1:40–52, 1964.
2. Wepman, J. *Auditory Discrimination Test*. Chicago: Language Research Associates, 1958.

CHAPTER 14

1. Cole, M., and Kraft, M. B. "Specific Learning Disability," *Cortex*, 1:302–313, 1964.

CHAPTER 15

1. Durrell, Donald D. *Improving Reading Instruction*. New York: World Book, 1956, p. 349.
2. *Ibid.*, pp. 352–353.
3. Mergentine, Charlotte. *You and Your Child's Reading, A Practical Guide for Parents*. New York: Harcourt, Brace and World, 1963, p. 25.

CHAPTER 16

1. Orton, J. L., in *The Disabled Reader,* John Money and Gilbert Schiffman, editors. Baltimore: Johns Hopkins University Press, 1966, p. 144.
2. Frostig, M., and Horne, D. *The Frostig Program for the Development of Visual Perception*. Chicago: Follett, 1964.
3. Kephart, N. *The Slow Learner in the Classroom*. Columbus: Charles E. Merrill, 1960.

CHAPTER 17

1. Gibson, Eleanor J., *op. cit.*, p. 1066.
2. Vernon, M. D. *Backwardness in Reading, op. cit.*, p. 1.

Suggested Additional Reading

Language and Psychology

BROWN, ROGER. *Words and Things*. Glencoe, Ill.: The Free Press, 1958.

GREGORY, R. L. *Eye and Brain, The Psychology of Seeing*. New York: McGraw-Hill, 1966.

HEBB, D. O. *The Organization of Behavior*. New York: John Wiley & Sons, 1949.

KOPPITZ, ELIZABETH M. *The Bender-Gestalt Test for Young Children*. New York: Grune & Stratton, 1964.

LAIRD, CHARLTON. *The Miracle of Language*. New York: Fawcett Books.

LASHLEY, K. S. *Brain Mechanisms and Intelligence*. New York: Hafner, 1964 (reprint).

VERNON, M. D. *A Further Study of Visual Perception*. Cambridge: Cambridge University Press, 1952.

Neurophysiology and Neurology

CRITCHLEY, MACDONALD. The Parietal Lobes. New York: Hafner, 1966 (reprint).

GROCH, JUDITH. *You and Your Brain*. New York: Harper & Row, 1963.

Handbook of Physiology. Section 1: Neurophysiology. Washington, D.C.: American Physiological Society, 1960 (especially Chapters 59–69, Volume 3).

MAGOUN, H. W. *The Waking Brain*. Springfield, Ill.: Charles C. Thomas, 1963.

PENFIELD, WILDER, and LAMAR ROBERTS. *Speech and Brain Mechanisms*. Princeton, N.J.: Princeton University Press, 1959.

WALTER, W. GREY. *The Living Brain*. New York: W. W. Norton, 1963.

Dyslexia

CRITCHLEY, MACDONALD. *Developmental Dyslexia*. Springfield, Ill.: Charles C. Thomas, 1964.

FLOWER, RICHARD M., HELEN F. GOFMAN and LUCIE I. LAWSON, editors. *Reading Disorders*. Philadelphia: F. A. Davis, 1965.

HALGREN, B. "Specific Dyslexia (Congenital Word-Blindness): A Clinical and Genetic Study," *Acta Psychiatrica et Neurologica Scandinavica,* Supplement 65, 1950.

HERMANN, KNUD. *Reading Disability: A Medical Study of Word-Blindness and Related Handicaps*. Springfield, Ill.: Charles C. Thomas, 1959.

MONEY, JOHN, ed. *Reading Disability: Progress and Research Needs in Dyslexia*. Baltimore, Md.: Johns Hopkins University Press, 1962.

MONEY, JOHN, and GILBERT SCHIFFMAN, eds. *The Disabled Reader*. Baltimore, Md.: Johns Hopkins University Press, 1966.

VERNON, M. D. *Backwardness in Reading*. Cambridge: Cambridge University Press, 1960.

Index